The Rainforest Medicinal Plant Guide Series

CAMU CAMU

(Myrciaria dubia)

NATURE'S SECRET
FOR DISEASE PREVENTION

I0135256

LESLIE TAYLOR, ND

Bestselling Author of *The Healing Power of Rainforest Herbs*

Rain-Tree
Publishers

The information and advice contained in this book are based upon the research and the professional experiences of the author, and are not intended as a substitute for consulting with a healthcare professional. The publisher and author are not responsible for any adverse effects or consequences resulting from the use of any of the suggestions discussed in this book. All matters pertaining to your physical health, including your diet and supplement routine, should be supervised by a healthcare professional who can provide medical care that is tailored to meet your individual needs.

Published by
Rain-Tree Publishers
Bullard, Texas 75757
www.rain-tree.com

ISBN: 978-1-7346847-3-5

Cover and Interior Production by Gary A. Rosenberg
www.thebookcouple.com

About the Rainforest Medicinal Plant Guide Series

This book is part of Leslie Taylor's Rainforest Medicinal Plant Guide series featuring the important medicinal plants of the rainforest that she has studied and used for more than 20 years. These guides provide factual, scientific, and vital information on how to use these powerful medicinal plants effectively to improve your health.

The author sells no herbal supplements or products other than books. The books in this series do not promote any specific brands or herbal supplement products. These definitive plant guides concern the plants and their researched effective actions and uses. The information in these guides is more extensive, complete, and unbiased than natural product companies who sell these plants as supplements can provide.

More information on Leslie Taylor's background, knowledge, and experience can be found on the Rain-Tree website (www.rain-tree.com/author.htm) See the Rain-Tree Publishers book page (www.rain-tree.com/books.htm) to learn when new plant guides in the series are released.

Contents

Introduction

Camu camu is a superfruit from the Amazon rainforest that is the richest source of vitamin C on the planet. However, as this book will explain, camu camu is so much more than just this one vital vitamin. Camu camu not only provides a full complement of vitamins, minerals, omega-3 and omega-6 fatty acids, and a therapeutic amount of potassium but also contains an exorbitant amount of natural plant compounds called polyphenols that naturally occur in many fruits and vegetables.

The natural health industry has been promoting various superfruits, fruit extract supplements, and fruit powders for many years for the many health benefits they provide—the majority of which come from their polyphenol content. North American and temperate-climate fruits that fall into the superfruit category include cranberries, goji berries, blueberries, grapes, pomegranates, mulberries, raspberries, strawberries, and blackberries. These fruits are all showing up in functional foods and beverages. However, there's a widely popular and growing market for tropical superfruit products. Tropical fruits such as camu camu, acai, noni, maqui, acerola, graviola, cherimoya, cupuacu, passion fruit, guava, lucuma, and others contain many more polyphenols than temperate-climate fruits, and wild-harvested tropical fruits have the highest level of all.

One of the many benefits polyphenols deliver is to provide strong antioxidant actions, which offer a wide array of health and disease-prevention benefits. The important information revealed in this book is that camu camu provides higher vitamin C (which has strong antioxidant actions) and more antioxidant polyphenols than any other known fruit in North or South America. New research also indicates that camu camu provides better antioxidant actions than all other fruits as well. No other fruit compares to the combination of very high vitamin C with very high polyphenol levels that camu camu delivers.

Health experts (and product marketers) tout super-fruits as nutrient-packed foods that can do everything from increase your energy, help you lose weight, and reduce aging to protect you from cancer, heart disease, diabetes, and other life-threatening illnesses. This book will help you, the consumer, separate the scientific facts from the marketing hype in the marketplace, learn which of these health claims are possible or probable, and how specifically polyphenols work to achieve these benefits. This book will also help you understand the actual studies conducted on camu camu and fruit polyphenols in general.

Introduction

The goal of this book is to finally explain that while our immune system protects us from infectious diseases and injuries, the main system in our bodies that protects us from chronic disease is our natural built-in antioxidant system, which is supposed to keep free radicals at healthy levels. You'll also learn:

❑ What causes this system to falter or fail.

❑ How our diets play a role in the health of our antioxidant system.

❑ What leading causes increase free radicals in our bodies and strain the system.

❑ What kind of cellular damage and deregulations are caused when this system falters or fails.

❑ What diseases and conditions we are at greater risk of developing when we have a faltering or failing antioxidant system.

❑ How to heal and repair this system and restore its ability to protect us from chronic disease.

Over the last year, I have been studying more than 1,000 polyphenol plant compounds and reading a huge number of clinical studies and published research on them. The amount of research on these important compounds is increasing daily with more than 10,000 studies on polyphenols published in just the last five years. New research on the actions and mechanisms of polyphenols, their effective dosages, and which plants and fruits contain enough to be therapeutic hold important information for the health and wellness of the planet. The recent growth in the knowledge of free radicals and plant-based polyphenols is producing a medical revolution that promises a new age of health and disease management in the research world. New drugs are on the horizon for the treatment of chronic diseases based on this research. However, polyphenols have surfaced in this new research as effective therapies for both new treatments and the prevention of many chronic diseases, and these are available to us now.

We used to get plenty of naturally occurring plant polyphenols in the fresh fruits and vegetables in our diet, but sadly, for far too many of us, that has become part of our past. Recent research reports that the main polyphenols in the average American diet now comes from coffee, chocolate, and wine. Fruit polyphenols are in fourth place, and vegetable-derived polyphenols comes in dead last.

New research confirms that the lack of polyphenols, which help keep our built-in antioxidant systems in good health, in our current diets has directly contributed to the rising number of preventable and chronic diseases our society is currently faced with. Almost half of the population now has some type of metabolic disease, which can lead to type 2 diabetes down the road. Half of Americans now have some sort of heart disease, fed by the alarming rates of hypertension (high blood pressure) reported today. And, shockingly, almost half the population is now overweight or obese, and those numbers continue to rise. This book will tell you how the failing antioxidant systems of Americans are contributing to the creation and progression of these three chronic diseases and many more, as well as how to turn the tide and jump-start your natural disease-prevention processes again.

After reviewing all the new research on polyphenols and camu camu and studying the specific polyphenols and the amounts provided in the fruit, I believe that camu camu's highest and best use to positively affect our health is by preventing these chronic diseases. If you choose to try camu camu for these purposes, this book provides vital information in a comprehensive consumer guide about the camu camu products available in the marketplace, how to choose the best product, and what dosages are most beneficial. Not all camu camu products are the equal (and some contain up to 87 percent less polyphenols!), and this book will tell you why and how to make informed choices when purchasing a camu camu (or any superfruit) supplement. You may not be able to find this in-depth information elsewhere, especially from an unbiased and reliable source that isn't trying to sell you their product.

I hope this book helps you find understanding and solutions to avoid many of the preventable diseases discussed in this book. Simple and natural health solutions such as these shouldn't be kept a secret but should be widely shared to lower our healthcare costs while benefiting our overall health and quality of life.

CHAPTER 1

What Is Camu camu?

Camu camu is a small tree or shrub found throughout the Amazon rainforest. Its scientific name is *Myrciaria dubia,* and it belongs in the large or *Myrtaceae* (myrtle) plant family. The myrtle family contains about 150 genera and 3,300 species of trees and shrubs. Its members are widely distributed in the tropics and include several well-known fruits and spices such as guava fruit as well as allspice, cloves, and eucalyptus. Many myrtle plants are cultivated around the world in the tropics as ornamentals and for the production of timber, oil, gum, tannin, resin, spices, and fruits.

Camu camu is indigenous to the Amazon rainforest where it grows naturally in seasonally flooded areas along rivers and oxbow lakes. Large stands of camu camu are a common sight along the banks of the Amazon and Ucayali rivers in Peru. The plant grows to a height of four to eight feet and has medium-sized green leaves with a leathery appearance. The plant produces round, dark reddish-purple fruits, which look similar to grapes, that are between one half to an inch in diameter (1 to 3 centimeters). The fruits start out green and develop their dark reddish-purple color from the bottom up as they ripen. Partially ripe fruits often have greenish-yellow shoulders with a dark-red bottom. Usually, camu camu fruit is wild harvested in the Amazon rainforest in canoes because the fruits mature at high-water or flooding season, which lasts four to five months out of the year. The plant produces one crop of fruit annually; however, the plants must be four to five years old before they bear fruit.

Camu camu fruits are actually a type of berry. Inside is a juicy, soft, very pale-yellow flesh and one to four large seeds. It is rarely eaten out of hand, as it tastes very sour with a bit of an odd aftertaste. In the tropics where it grows, it is usually made into juices, jellies, sauces, ice cream, and other sweetened foods and beverages to counteract its very tart taste.

Camu camu is currently an important and promising economic fruit species grown in the Peruvian Amazon, as well as in Brazil, Colombia, and Bolivia. The fruit is valued for its high content of vitamin C, which is higher than any other fruit. Large plantations have been established only in the last 15 years; however, a substantial part of the production of camu camu in South America is still obtained by collecting fruits from the wild. New studies are underway in Brazil aimed at improving the quality/ yield of the fruit production, at adapting the plant to firm land thus increasing possible plantation areas and regions, and also making the fruit viable for consumption in regions where it is not cultivated.

Tribal and Herbal Medicine Uses

Camu camu fruit was never documented as a traditional herbal remedy for any condition in the Amazon region before a market was created for it in the United States and Japan. In fact, it wasn't even widely eaten as a fruit by the indigenous people due to its sour, acidic taste. However, the leaves and bark of the camu camu shrub have been used by rainforest inhabitants as a natural remedy for malaria, parasitic infections, and other medicinal purposes for hundreds of years. Today, many camu camu fruit products, sweetened juices, and even ice creams and popsicles can be found in the larger cities and towns in the Brazilian and Peruvian Amazon regions, promoting the same health benefits as are now being promoted here as a superfruit.

Natural Compounds and Nutritional Value

Camu camu fruit has the highest recorded amount of natural vitamin C known on the planet in a fruit. Oranges provide 500 to 4,000 ppm (parts per million) vitamin C, or ascorbic acid; acerola, another tropical fruit, has tested in the range of 16,000 to 172,000 ppm. Camu camu provides up to 500,000 ppm, or about 2 grams of vitamin C per 100 grams (about 3.5 ounces) of fresh fruit. Special cultivars developed in Brazil have higher levels of vitamin C; their camu camu fruit has 3 to 5 grams of vitamin C in 100 grams of fresh fruit. In comparison to oranges, camu

camu provides up to 100 times more vitamin C, 10 times more iron, 3 times more niacin, 2 times more riboflavin, and 1.5 times more phosphorus.

Camu camu fruits are good source of minerals, including potassium, calcium, zinc, magnesium, manganese, and copper. Camu camu fruits also contain different types of amino acids such as serine, valine, leucine, glutamate, 4-aminobutanoate, proline, phenylalanine, threonine, and alanine. Different organic acids such as citric acid, isocitric acid, and malic acid also have been identified in camu camu fruits. In addition, it also contains different kinds of omega-3 and omega-6 fatty acids, mainly stearic, linoleic, oleic, linolenic, tricosanoic, eicosadienoic acids. In addition, there are 21 volatile compounds found in camu camu fruits. Some of these minerals (especially potassium) and other constituents aid in the absorption and uptake of the high amount of vitamin C the fruit provides. Studies indicate that absorption and uptake of vitamin C is much higher in camu camu due to these other constituents than taking a synthetic single-chemical vitamin C supplement.

The nutritional value of camu camu has earned its place in the functional food "superfruit" category in the natural products market along other superfruits such as noni, açai, goji berry, acerola, and graviola fruits.

As with any vitamin C–rich fruit, the time between harvesting and consumption is crucial; the fruit may lose up to a quarter of its vitamin C content in less than a month (even if frozen). Even with this loss, camu camu still has an edge over all other challengers in the super-fruit category.

While vitamin C is known to be a powerful antioxidant (a substance that can scavenge free radicals), camu

FOOD VALUE OF CAMU CAMU FRUIT PER 100 GRAMS FRESH WEIGHT	
Water	94.1 g
Calories	17
Protein	400 mg
Lipids (fatty acids)	20 mg
Calcium	15.7 mg
Iron	0.53 mg
Magnesium	12.4 mg
Manganese	2.1 mg
Phosphorus	2.83 mg
Polyphenols	1,196 mg
Potassium	83.8 mg
Carotenoids	355 mcg
Thiamine	1.7 mg
Riboflavin	0.04 mg
Niacin	6 mg
Vitamin C	2,000 mg
Vitamin A	2.45 mg
Zinc	0.36 mg

camu fruits are a major source of bioactive compounds called polyphenols. These include flavonoids, phenolic acids, tannins, stilbenes, and lignans, which are generated in plants as a part their own unique and complicated chemical defense mechanism to reduce oxidative stress and heal damage from fungi and bacteria, soil viruses, intense heat and light, and to recover from insect predation. These polyphenol compounds can possess four to five times the antioxidant power as vitamins C and E. Much more information on polyphenols can be found in chapters 4 and 5.

The main active chemicals in camu camu that have been correlated with the fruit's biological activities are those that are delivered in high amounts, including ellagitannins, ellagic acid, quercetin, and myricetin. Almost half of camu camu's polyphenols are some form of ellagic acid. Ellagic acid and the metabolites it forms in plants and humans are well studied. This powerful polyphenol is mostly found in red, blue, and purple fruits and some nuts. Thus far, camu camu has been shown to deliver more ellagic acid than many other fruit supplements that are sold for their biological actions related to ellagic acid, including pomegranate, grapeseed, blueberry, blackberry, and mulberry.

Camu camu not only provides the highest amount of vitamin C of all superfruits, it also contains the highest amount of beneficial polyphenol compounds. If you compare the polyphenols in other superfruits sold in the marketplace that tout the health benefits of their polyphenols (for disease prevention, anti-aging, weight-loss, inflammation, etc.), camu camu beats them all. The main superfruits touted for their beneficial polyphenols include noni, açai, goji berry, and acerola. Research published in 2018 tested all these superfruits for polyphenols and vitamin C and indicated the following results (in 100 grams fresh/10 grams of dried fruit), which should earn camu camu the designation of a *super* superfruit.

Fruit	Polyphenols	Vitamin C
Camu Camu	1,196 mg	1,882 mg
Açai	529 mg	84 mg
Acerola	855 mg	1,350 mg
Goji berry	268 mg	49 mg
Noni	748 mg	76 mg

In addition to the vitamins and minerals mentioned earlier, camu camu contains 4-o-methylellagic-acid, 4-terpinol, alanine, all-trans-lutein, alpha-carotene, alpha-fenchene, alpha-phellandrene, alpha-pinene, alpha-rhamnopyranosyl-ellagic-acid, alpha-terpinene, beta-caryophyllene, beta-carotene, beta-myrcene, beta-phellandrene, beta-pinene, camphene, car-3-ene, castalagin, casuarinin, celphinidin-3-glucoside, cis-neoxanthin, citrate, citric acid, chlorogenic acid, cyanidin, cyanidin-3-glucoside, cyanidin-3-O-glucoside, d-limonene, dehydroascorbic acid, delphinidin,

delphinidin-3-glucoside, di-hexahydroxydiphenoyl glucose, ellagic acid, ellagic acid glycosides, ellagic acid deoxyhexoside, ellagic acid pentoside, ellagic acid hexoside, eucalyptol, ellagitannins, eriodictyol, epicatechin, fenchol, gallic acid, gallotannins, gamma-terpinene, grandinin, humulene, isocitric acid, isomyrtucommulone B, isorhamnetin, kaempferol, leucine, lutein, luteoxanthin, malate, 1-methyl malate, 1,4-dimethyl malate, malic acid, malvidin, myrciarone A & B, myricetin, myricetin-3-O-hexoside, myricetin-3-O-pentoside, naringenin, neoxanthin, p-cymene, pelargonidin, peonidin, petunidin, phenylalanine, prolene, quercetin, quercetin-3-O-hexoside, quercetin-3-O-pentoside, quercitrin, rhodomyrtone, rutin, serine, stachyurin, syringic acid, tartrate, terpinolene, threonine, valine, vescalagin, violaxanthins, and zeaxanthin.

I've used the word *antioxidant* several times in this chapter to describe various compounds in camu camu. Before we go much farther, I want to make sure you really know what an antioxidant is and how it is capable of fighting free radicals, and even what a free radical really is. The next chapter will tell you more about antioxidants, free radicals, and how vitamin C and other compounds found in camu camu will help you maintain the delicate balance you need for healthy antioxidant levels and why that is so important.

CHAPTER 2

Free Radicals
and Antioxidants

The average American typically has some kind of basic knowledge (usually from advertisements) that "antioxidants fight free radicals," but most are unaware of exactly what a free radical is, why they need fighting, and how antioxidants work to "quench" or fight them. This chapter will explain the main types of free radicals, how they cause cellular damage, cellular dysfunction, and resulting illness, and the different ways specialized natural plant compounds with antioxidant actions (as well as vitamin C) can effectively reduce the number of free radicals in your body to promote health and avoid disease. Some of the powerful natural antioxidants discussed in this chapter can also stop cells from being damaged by free radicals and even help repair the damage they've already caused.

What Is a Free Radical?

There are two main types of free radicals: reactive oxygen species (ROS) and reactive nitrogen species (RNS). These substances are reactive because they are missing an electron. Our bodies are an oxygen-based system, as is most all life on the planet. Oxygen is an element indispensable for life. However, inside the body, some oxygen, with the help of a catalyst, splits into single atoms with unpaired electrons. Electrons like to be in pairs, so these atoms, called free radicals, scavenge the body for other electrons so they can become a pair. As they travel through the body in search of a new electron, they cause damage to cells, proteins, and DNA, and interrupt or change cellular signaling through a process called oxidation.

Consider what happens when you put a piece of untreated and unprotected metal outside in the elements or simply expose it to oxygen. Over time, the metal begins to rust. This rusting process is actually the oxidation of the metal—the chemical reaction of the metal to oxygen. ROS inside the body creates the same sort of rust-like reaction and damage as it comes into contact with unprotected cells. As another example: when the fats or oils we use to cook with are exposed to too much oxygen, over time they become rancid. The rancidity is actually oxidation of the fat molecules. When fat molecules (called lipids) in our bodies are exposed to too much ROS, they also rust or become rancid in a similar manner. For this reason, the oxygen-based free radicals (ROS) are much more damaging to our bodies, are the subject of much more research, are linked to many more diseases and conditions, and are what we will focus on in this book.

Free radicals, and specifically ROS, are a way of life.

ROS are formed as a natural byproduct of the normal metabolism of oxygen, and they even play important roles in how cells communicate (called cellular signaling). Basically, free radicals are a byproduct of many different chemical processes going on simultaneously inside our wonderfully complex biochemical-driven bodies.

In addition to metabolizing oxygen, another large source of free radicals produced inside our bodies is the natural chemical process of how we metabolize our foods. Turning food into the cellular energy that all our cells need to function and even to survive is a complex biochemical process. Free radicals are waste products generated from various chemical reactions that occur in this natural food metabolism process. Therefore, how much we eat and what we eat can be significant factors that raise our ROS levels.

ROS are created inside our bodies through these natural processes, and catalyst substances in our environment can create even more ROS. External catalysts that generate free radicals can be found in the food we eat, the medicines we take, the air we breathe, and the water we drink. These substances include fried foods, high-fructose sugars, alcohol, tobacco smoke, pesticides, exposure to X-rays, chemicals and environmental toxins, and air and water pollutants. All these substances can significantly raise the levels of ROS and free radicals in our bodies to unhealthy levels, which results in oxidative stress. The levels of internally produced free radical also increase from immune cell activation, inflammation, mental stress, excessive exercise, ischemia, infection, cancer, aging, diabetes, and obesity, which takes us over the edge of balance and into the state of oxidative stress. ROS can also provoke inappropriate or overexpressed immune responses and cause autoimmune conditions, activate cancer genes, mutate healthy cells into cancerous ones, and greatly increase cellular-aging processes.

What Is an Antioxidant?

In the simplest of terms, the most basic definition of an antioxidant is a substance or molecule that lends one of its own electrons to a free radical that is seeking one to make a pair. When the free radical has a new set of paired electrons, it becomes a stable molecule and is no longer reactive and causing cell damage. Remember, free radicals are radical because they are missing an electron. This process of an antioxidant lending an electron is usually called "quenching free radicals."

Our Built-In Antioxidant System

Because ROS generation is a natural process, our bodies have a natural built-in antioxidant system that is supposed to disable these free radicals as they are created and keep them at healthy levels. This is a perfect example of one of the amazing ways our bodies maintain their delicate balance. Through other biochemical processes, our bodies produce chemicals that are the main antioxidants that make up our built-in antioxidant system. These include chemical enzymes called superoxide dismutase (SOD), catalase, glutathione peroxidase, and glutathione reductase, which are considered our first line of defense.

We also produce other substances that are non-enzyme antioxidants that participate in our built-in antioxidant system. These include chemicals we produce inside our bodies (and some of which are also sold as dietary supplements) such as lipoic acid, glutathione, L-arginine, coenzyme Q10, melatonin, uric acid, bilirubin, metal-chelating proteins, transferrin, and others.

Vitamin and Mineral Antioxidants

While these natural built-in antioxidants are main players in our antioxidant system, they need help from various vitamins and minerals that aid in the biochemical process to produce them, activate them, and help them do their job. These include vitamins A, E, and C, which we're supposed to be getting from the foods we eat. These three vitamins are the subject of thousands of studies on their antioxidant actions and the roles they play in the body and within our antioxidant system. Of these three vitamin antioxidants, vitamin C has been shown to be the most important to the system. And, as with many antioxidants, the combination of vitamin C with either A or E has shown to have higher antioxidant actions in much of the vitamin research. Vitamin C is also uniquely able to lend not one, but two of its electrons to free radicals. In addition, as discussed in the next chapter, vitamin C plays an essential role for our natural enzyme antioxidants to be produced inside the body and for them to do their job efficiently.

Also necessary to support our antioxidant system and its enzymes are the minerals selenium, manganese, copper, and zinc. These minerals play roles in the production and/or actions of our natural enzymes that fight free radicals. In fact, some of these minerals are capable of binding together with our enzymes, which increases their antioxidant actions and effects.

Plant Antioxidants

Plants, like humans, need oxygen to survive, and they also create their own species of reactive oxygen molecules (ROS) during their metabolism of the oxygen they breathe. For this reason, plants produce natural antioxidants in their cellular processes to keep ROS in check and at healthy levels, just as we do. These antioxidant plant chemicals are also an important component in a plant's built-in defense mechanisms (much like our immune system) that protect the plants from damage and stress of too much or too little rainfall/moisture, too much or too little sunlight, toxic metals and chemicals in their soil, high heat, intense sunlight, high humidity, and other negative growing factors. These natural plant antioxidant compounds also help heal the damage from browsing animals and insects chewing on them (the equivalent of wounds in humans) and help plants recover from various bacteria, mold, fungi, and plant viruses that damage them. In fact, many plant antioxidants are dually antioxidant and antimicrobial—capable of killing these bacteria and fungi species that try to harm them. Because plants are rooted to the ground and cannot flee from danger like we can, they create wonderfully complex biochemical defense mechanisms to fight those dangers and factors that might harm or kill them.

In addition to lending electrons, plant antioxidants can suppress the formation of ROS by inhibiting certain enzymes involved in their production. Plant antioxidants can also trigger the body's natural production of antioxidants and send them to cells that are being damaged by oxidative stress. Much as chemical messengers signal the immune system to send healing agents to the site of an injury, plant antioxidants signal the body's antioxidant system to send healing antioxidants to the site of oxidative stress, as well as encourage the production of more body-produced antioxidant chemicals.

Lastly, there are various metals in our bodies—including the iron circulating in our blood—that can oxidize and damage cells, much as ROS does. Some strong plant antioxidants, like those found in camu camu, are capable of interacting with these metals and converting the body's metal pro-oxidants into stable products, much as they stabilize or neutralize free radicals, reducing oxidative stress.

Polyphenol Antioxidants

The main and most effective antioxidants found in plants fall into a category of well-researched plant compounds called polyphenols. Scientists have long known that the polyphenols in plants can benefit humans in many of same ways they benefit, protect, and heal plants. Polyphenols, which include the subcategories of phenolic acids and flavonoids, are the subject of a huge amount of research. More than 10,000 studies on plant polyphenols have been published in just the last five years. Not only do they have very strong antioxidant actions, but because they were uniquely created to help plants heal and repair damage, their actions in humans result in these antioxidants working in different ways than vitamin antioxidants and our own natural enzyme antioxidants, which are mainly quenching free radicals through electron sharing. The healing power of these polyphenols to positively affect our health is incredible, and thankfully more health-conscious consumers are learning of their many benefits.

Remember when coffee was once supposed to be bad for you and doctors told you to avoid it, mainly because of the heart-stimulant actions of caffeine? Then, suddenly, it was good for you. The same thing happened with chocolate and wine, which once were supposed to be avoided and are now considered almost health foods. What happened? It was all the new research on the powerful health benefits of polyphenols. Coffee, chocolate (especially dark chocolate), and wine (mostly red wine) are all significant sources of these powerful healing polyphenols. That polyphenols can overcome the negative effects of the caffeine in coffee, the high fat and calories in chocolate, and the alcohol content in wine, and still provide a net effect that is beneficial to our health speaks to the real power of these polyphenols.

In addition to coffee, wine, and chocolate, it is the fruits and vegetables in our diets that are our main source of healthy polyphenols. Polyphenols are also found in the oils of plant seeds and fruit seeds, and this is one of the reasons why olive oil is now widely consumed as a "healthy oil"—it is rich in polyphenols. The polyphenol content of the foods we eat vary widely based on many factors. And like vitamin C, some powerful polyphenols are water soluble and are very sensitive to heat. The high heat generated in cooking fruits and vegetables can significantly lower the polyphenol content, which is why many nutritionists recommend having lots of raw fruits and veggies in our diets—it's all about the powerful and beneficial polyphenols in these raw foods. Much more information on polyphenols are found in chapter 4.

Summary

In a perfect world, we'd be getting all the vitamins, minerals, plant antioxidants, and other vital nutrients we need from the foods we eat. We'd avoid foods that generate extra free radicals, and we'd maintain a healthy weight and a healthy antioxidant system as a result. More important, in doing so, we'd be providing all the necessary nutrients all these complicated biochemical processes need that are humming along silently behind the scenes—all of which keep us healthy and avoiding problems and diseases.

But let's face it. We don't live in a perfect world, and we are merely imperfect humans. That kind of scenario just doesn't describe the average American and or even the average human. I think that's why "food supplements" and "dietary supplements" were first created and related to that kind of terminology. Many of these products really *are* supplementing our diets with the necessary food nutrients that are missing from the foods we eat. Other dietary supplements are helping to overcome the problems from too many of the less-than-healthy foods and lifestyle choices we can't seem to give up.

This is why getting our daily needs of vitamin C is much better when it comes from a whole food source like camu camu. Camu camu contains a host of other beneficial natural plant compounds, including polyphenols, which naturally occur in the foods we're supposed to be eating in our daily diet. In addition to polyphenols, camu camu contains fatty acids, carotenoids, and other plant compounds with effective antioxidant effects. These are the compounds that aid in the absorption and uptake of the vitamins and minerals in the fruit, provide synergistic actions to help vitamin C be a better antioxidant, and provide added antioxidant actions as well as host of other benefits and actions all on their own.

A single chemical, synthetically made ascorbic acid supplement just doesn't compare. While the vitamin C content may be equal between a synthetic vitamin C supplement and an camu camu supplement, with camu camu, you get so much more than just vitamin C. That being said, it is still always better to get the antioxidants we need from a diet rich in fruits and vegetables rather than from supplements. When we can't, a high quality camu camu supplement is a wonderful healthy alternative.

While vitamin C is one of the better known and researched natural antioxidants, it also provides many other functions for health, which will be discussed in the next chapter. You will learn why it is an essential vitamin required for many cellular functions for optimal health.

CHAPTER 3

The Health Benefits of Vitamin C

Vitamin C is essential for life, and yet, humans are among just a few types of mammals that cannot produce it within their bodies. Vitamin C must be obtained through our diet. Vitamin C, also known as ascorbic acid, isn't just an antioxidant. It is necessary for the growth, development, and repair of all body tissues. It's involved in many bodily functions, including formation of collagen, absorption of iron, production of immune system cells to fight infection, wound healing, and the maintenance of cartilage, bones, and teeth. In fact, this essential vitamin can be found residing in almost all the cells in our body in tiny amounts.

Vitamin C is an integral part of our built-in antioxidant system, including acting as a cofactor to support other natural antioxidant compounds our bodies produce that keep free radicals in check and at healthy levels. Vitamin C is the most abundant water-soluble vitamin antioxidant in our blood and tissues, and one of the most famous antioxidant supplements. It has been linked to many impressive health benefits, such as boosting over-all natural antioxidant levels, reducing blood pressure, reducing heart disease risk, protecting against gout attacks, improving iron absorption, boosting immunity, reducing dementia risk, and reducing cancer risk.

We have known about the importance of vitamin C for centuries. Deficient amounts of this essential vitamin cause a disease called scurvy. The word *scurvy* was first recorded in an English seaman's record in 1589. Sailors on long voyages with a lack of vitamin C–rich fresh fruits and vegetables in their diets were especially prone to developing this dreaded disease. It is estimated that more than 1 million sailors died during the seventeenth and eighteenth centuries due to scurvy.

The U.S. recommended dietary allowance (RDA) for vitamin C is 75 milligrams for women and 90 milligrams for men. Just one camu camu fruit would more than sat-isfy the RDA. However, this is generally regarded by most as the minimum amount necessary to avoid deficiencies. Much higher dosages of vitamin C are considered more therapeutic and beneficial by many natural health prac-titioners, and research has confirmed many benefits at higher-than-RDA dosages.

As vitamin C is water-soluble, it is not stored in the body, and therefore, there are few risks related to over-consumption. Whatever is not used by the body is simply excreted through urine. Humans also have a very small capacity for storing vitamin C; we can only hold about a thirty-day supply. Therefore, it is absolutely necessary to get our vitamin C from external dietary sources on a daily basis.

The Main Benefits and Actions of Vitamin C

The extensive research on vitamin C reveals the important health benefits discussed next. (See the reference section for a list of the research detailed.)

A Natural Antioxidant to Fight Free Radicals

Vitamin C is probably one of the best known and widely studied natural antioxidants. It has been the subject of human and animal studies over many years and well documented to reduce or neutralize free radicals and aids other natural antioxidants we produce to do their job more effectively. Vitamin C is typically used as a gold standard to compare the antioxidant abilities of other substances that are studied in several antioxidant laboratory tests.

Enhances Immune Function

One of the main reasons people take vitamin C supplements is to boost their immunity. The human immune system produces white blood cells called phagocytes. *Phagocytosis* is a medical term that describes the ingestion and destruction of bacteria, viruses, and other foreign invaders by these phagocytes. This is the chief defense mechanism of the human body against infection—our immune system's main role. The ability of phagocytes to carry out these activities has been shown to be associated with the presence of vitamin C in white blood cells. Vitamin C plays an important role in aiding these immune cells to function normally and kill micro-organisms. Research indicates that raising levels of vitamin C in the body increases phagocytosis and helps the body fight infections more effectively. It has also been established through research to actually encourage the production of phagocytes and other white blood cells known as lymphocytes that also enhance immune function response. Moreover, vitamin C is helpful to strengthen the skin's immune defense system and helps wounds heal faster.

Promotes Collagen Production

Most people are aware that one of the main reasons our skin develops wrinkles as we age is a gradual loss of collagen in our skin. There is certainly no shortage of skin-care potions marketed to women to retard skin aging and decrease wrinkles by supposedly increasing skin collagen. Many of these anti-wrinkle potions even contain natural or synthetic vitamin C. However, you might be surprised to learn that collagen is about much more than just wrinkles. Collagen is actually the structural glue that holds us together as human beings. Collagen is the most abundant protein in mammals, making up from 25 to 35 percent of the whole-body protein content. It's the basic building block of all connective tissue that builds and strengthens not only skin, but teeth, bones, blood vessels, ligaments, and tendons as well.

Vitamin C is necessary to create collagen in our bodies in several different ways. Mostly, it is a cofactor (helper) for several important enzymes that actually make collagen. Without adequate vitamin C, these enzymes can't do their job and collagen production slows down. Most of the symptoms and ill effects of the vitamin C–deficient disease, scurvy, is due to a significant loss of collagen. Scurvy causes subcutaneous bleeding and bruising (due to weak blood vessels), poor wound healing (from poor skin collagen and immune function), joint pain and swelling (weak cartilage and ligaments), and thin hair and tooth loss (from a lack of collagen in those structures). The fatigue well noted in scurvy may well come from other enzymes that require vitamin C to produce L-carnitine. This is a molecule that converts fat into energy. Without enough of this enzyme, the body may not be able to burn fat, which will diminish fuel for energy production and cause fatigue as well as promote fat accumulation and weight gain.

Therefore, while promoting collagen production may well help keep our skin looking younger, it's hugely important to support the body's overall collagen production to keep bones, blood vessels, teeth, and the whole body strong. Making sure you have good vitamin C levels is necessary for this important aspect of wellness.

Promotes Healthy Aging

Researchers in Korea reported in 2015 that high dosages of vitamin C (1,250 milligrams daily) reduced the levels of advanced glycation end products (AGEs) in their human studies. AGEs are well documented to promote premature and regular cellular aging. They accumulate in the body (and skin) as we age and are a direct cause of many age-related chronic diseases and conditions. In addition, researchers examined links between nutrient intakes and skin aging in 4,025 women over age 40. They reported that higher vitamin C levels were associated with a lower likelihood of a wrinkled skin appearance, dryness of the skin, and a better skin-aging appearance. Taking vitamin C orally and using it topically has evidenced benefits to retard skin aging through the reduction of AGEs and oxidative stress, in addition to promoting collagen levels in the skin. In fact, it is the actual collagen in our skin that suffers the most damage from AGEs and free radicals, which causes the skin to age and wrinkle. See chapter 6 for more information on AGEs and the damage they cause, and how camu camu may prevent AGE formation, disable them, and/or reduce their damaging effects.

Improves Mood Disorders

Vitamin C is believed to be involved in anxiety, stress, depression, fatigue, and our overall mood state. A significant amount of vitamin C is stored in the brain and helps regulate brain function. It has been demonstrated in human clinical trials in adults, adolescents, and children that oral vitamin C supplementation (1 to 3 grams daily) can elevate mood as well as reduce depression, stress, and anxiety. And, once again, having low levels of vitamin C due to poor diets has been reported to increase the risk of developing these types of mood disorders in all age groups.

Memory and Neurodegenerative Disorders

Vitamin C has been shown to participate in many different neurochemical reactions involving electron transport. Neurons are known to use vitamin C for many different chemical and enzymatic reactions, including the synthesis of neurotransmitters and hormones. Norepinephrine is an essential neurotransmitter that controls attention and memories in our brains. It's also responsible for delivering our biochemical response to physical and emotional stress, and it's made with the help of vitamin C.

Recent research has reported that higher doses of vitamin C are beneficial for various degenerative brain conditions such as Parkinson's disease, Alzheimer's disease, dementia, age-related memory loss, and others. Most of these benefits are attributed to the antioxidant actions of vitamin C and its ability to relieve oxidative stress, which is well known to be elevated in the brain in these types of neurodegenerative disorders.

Furthermore, high vitamin C intake from food or supplements has been shown to have a protective effect on thinking and memory with age. See more information in chapter 5 on how free radicals can create oxidative stress in the brain to cause these disorders.

Helps Regulate Blood Pressure

The ability of vitamin C to help regulate blood pressure has been well documented. Researchers at Johns Hopkins School of Medicine analyzed 29 human studies and reported in 2012 that taking a vitamin C supplement (averaging 500 milligrams per day) can help lower blood pressure. It should be noted, however, that the drop in blood pressure levels in these studies were moderate and not strong enough to treat most hypertensive patients effectively as a stand-alone treatment. In people who had high blood pressure in these reviewed studies, systolic blood pressure (the top number in a reading) dropped by an average of nearly 5 points, while diastolic pressure (the bottom number) dropped by about 1.7 points. Once again, these benefits to modulate blood pressure are thought to be mainly attributed to the vitamin's antioxidant actions. The antioxidant activities of vitamin C may protect the lining of blood vessels from damage caused by oxidative stress and increase the availability of nitric oxide, a signaling molecule that helps relax arterial walls and reduce pressure.

Regulates Cholesterol and Prevents Clogged Arteries

Research reports that higher doses of vitamin C (1 to 3 grams daily) helps normalize and lower cholesterol levels. The antioxidant action of vitamin C also plays a role in preventing the oxidation of low-density lipoprotein (LDL) cholesterol. Oxidized LDL is one of the main components of arterial plaque. Having less oxidized LDL in our bloodstream helps prevent clogged arteries thereby naturally reducing the risk of heart diseases. As a result, many human studies report that consuming at least 500 milligrams of vitamin C daily may reduce the risk of heart disease. Additionally, research published in the *American Journal of Clinical Nutrition* found that those with the highest concentrations of vitamin C in their blood had a 42 percent lower stroke risk than those with the lowest concentrations.

Enhances Iron Absorption and Treats Anemia

Vitamin C supplementation has been used as a means of reducing iron deficiency and treating anemia as it aids in the absorption and uptake of iron from the diet. Vitamin C is able to convert plant-based sources of iron into a form that is easier for us to absorb. Research reports that taking just 100 milligrams of vitamin C may improve iron absorption by 67 percent. Researchers in China reported that a dose of just 50 milligrams daily effectively treated mild anemia in children as a stand-alone treatment.

Supports Male Fertility

Low vitamin C levels has been associated with male fertility problems. Vitamin C supplementation (at a minimum dosage of 500 milligrams daily) has been reported in several studies to enhance the production and mobility of sperm in both humans and animals. The fertility-enhancing action of vitamin C is mostly attributed to its antioxidant actions.

Benefits for Cold and Flu

Vitamin C has long been reported to be beneficial for colds and flu. Dosages from 2 to 4 grams and up to 8 grams daily have shown to ease symptoms of colds and flu and shorten the duration of infection. Lower dosages have shown little to no results in other research, which to some, makes the research seemingly inconsistent. However, if one compares the dosages used in all the research studies, it's clear this benefit is achieved with higher dosages. It's also possible that the immune system benefits discussed earlier that vitamin C increases phagocytosis plays a role in assisting the white blood cells to fight the infection more effectively. In fact, during the recent coronavirus outbreak in China, protocols were developed to treat hospitalized patients with high-dose vitamin C.

Benefits for Allergies and Asthma

Research reports people who took vitamin C regularly had fewer allergy problems, respiratory infections, and asthma attacks. A 1992 study found lower blood levels of histamine (which causes allergic reactions) in people who took 2 grams of vitamin C daily. In research conducted in Germany in 2018, high-dose vitamin C (intravenously) was reported to reduce allergy-related symptoms and act as an antihistamine.

Prevention of Glaucoma and Eye Diseases

Vitamin C has been shown to in several studies to lower intraocular pressure, which is elevated in glaucoma. Low levels of vitamin C has also been shown to increase the risk of developing glaucoma. Other research reports that vitamin C may provide benefits for age-related macular degeneration and cataracts. Most of the eye benefits reported for vitamin C are mainly attributed to the antioxidant actions of vitamin C and its ability to reduce oxidative stress and resulting damage in the eyes.

Adjunctive Support for Shingles

Shingles (a *Herpes zoster* infection) has been successfully treated with antioxidative substances like high-dose vitamin C for many years. Generally, vitamin C in high dosages, given orally or administered intravenously, has been shown in research to lessen the duration of the infection and reduce or prevent long-term nerve pain, which can persist after the infection. Antioxidants in general have been shown in research to protect nerves from oxidative stress and the damage it causes, which is a contributing factor in the nerve pain some people experience long after the virus causing the infection is gone.

Treats and Prevents Gout

Gout is an extremely painful condition caused by too much uric acid in body. Gout is actually a type of arthritis and occurs when excess uric acid crystalizes and deposits in the joints, causing pain and inflammation. Several human studies report that higher dosages of vitamin C (500 milligrams daily or more) can significantly lower uric acid levels and treat the condition, while other studies report lower dosages (100 to 300 milligrams daily) are beneficial in preventing future gout attacks. One study followed 46,994 healthy men over 20 years to see if vitamin C intake was linked to developing gout. Interestingly, their research revealed that people who took a vitamin C supplement had a 44 percent lower gout risk.

Cancer and Cancer Prevention

Over the past century, the notion that vitamin C can be used to treat cancer has generated much controversy. Vitamin C was first shown to be a potent, nontoxic, anticancer agent by Nobel Prize winner Linus Pauling in 1976. In his research, Pauling showed a 4.2 times longer survival time for terminal cancer patients who received 10 grams (10,000 milligrams) of intravenous vitamin C per day for 10 days, followed by 10 grams of oral vitamin C per day indefinitely. Subsequent research performed by others had some conflicts as well as different outcomes, and the use of vitamin C for cancer didn't fully catch on in mainstream medicine circles for many years.

However, new knowledge regarding how vitamin C works in the body and recent high-profile preclinical studies have revived interest in the utilization of high-dose vitamin C for cancer treatment. Studies have shown that intravenous vitamin C targets many of the mechanisms that cancer cells utilize for their survival and growth. The current mainstream thinking is that since the body's store of vitamin C is tightly controlled by several different built-in mechanisms, oral supplementation of the vitamin cannot achieve blood levels high enough that provide the ability to kill cancer cells. For this reason, most all human and animal research focusing on vitamin C and cancer today are using high dosages delivered intravenously. Intravenous vitamin C achieves blood concentration levels between 100 and 1,000 times higher than oral vitamin C can.

Cancer prevention, however, is a completely different story. Natural antioxidants (including vitamin C and other natural antioxidants found in camu camu) have demonstrated in a huge body of research over the years to be beneficial in reducing the risk of developing cancer. Most of this research confirms that having a healthy built-in antioxidant system is the best method to prevent cancer.

One of the most compelling cases I am aware of for using vitamin C for cancer is from a friend and colleague, James Templeton. He is a long-term survivor of stage-5 melanoma who used high-dose intravenous vitamin C in the Pauling protocol many years ago when it was still rather controversial. His new book, *I Used to Have Cancer*, is a heartfelt account of his journey to healing and explains how vitamin C was integral to his cure and why he still takes high dosages of this important vitamin for prevention and wellness.

The Bottom Line

Vitamin C has gained a great deal of attention, especially lately—and for good reason. A recent study published in *Seminars in Preventive and Alternative Medicine* looked at over 100 studies over 10 years which revealed a growing list of benefits of vitamin C. The lead researcher, Mark Moyad, MD, MPH, of the University of Michigan said in the publication: "Higher blood levels of vitamin C may be the ideal nutrition marker for overall health. The more we study vitamin C, the better our understanding of how diverse it is in protecting our health, from cardiovascular, cancer, stroke, eye health, [and] immunity to living longer." He also notes most of the benefits studied are achieved at higher dosages starting at 400 to 500 milligrams daily or higher.

Overall, vitamin C is linked to many impressive health benefits, and vitamin C supplements are a simple and cost-effective way to boost your vitamin C levels. With the rising number of Americans relying on processed, pre-prepared, and fast foods in their busy lives, lower nutritional levels, including low vitamin C levels, can be a result.

The recommended number of servings of fruits and vegetables is nine daily—a number most Americans struggle to meet. When you consider that vitamin C is heat sensitive and boiling or cooking can lower a food's nutritional value, including vitamin C levels, many people may be deficient in this essential vitamin without being aware of it. If you struggle to get enough natural vitamin C from the raw fruits and vegetables in your diet to maintain adequate nutrition, you should consider taking a vitamin C supplement.

Vitamin C Deficiencies

Smokers and low-income families are among those most at risk for vitamin C deficiencies. Regular alcohol consumption (and overconsumption) can also create vitamin C deficiencies. People (and especially children) with limited variety in their diets, people with malabsorption issues, and those with certain chronic diseases, long-lasting illnesses, and cancer may all experience vitamin C deficiencies. When illness strikes, the immune system responds naturally by increasing white blood cells to fight the illness. This can quickly deplete the body's store of vitamin C that these white blood cells require to do their job. If the illness is prolonged, vitamin C deficiency can result.

The first symptom of a vitamin C deficiency is unexplained fatigue. More subtle symptoms of vitamin C deficiencies (which can take months of chronic low levels to develop) include rough, bumpy skin, bruising easily, slow-healing wounds, painful or swollen joints, weak bones, bleeding gums, immune deficiencies, poor mood, thinning hair, and unexplained weight gain.

Camu Camu as a Solution

Whether you think you might have low levels of this important vitamin or you want to have optimal levels for the benefits detailed in this chapter, supplementing with camu camu for your vitamin C needs is an option health-conscious people are turning to. A significant amount of natural vitamin C is delivered along with a host of other beneficial vitamin, minerals, and natural plant compounds that facilitate greater absorption and utilization by all the different cells and biochemical processes that require vitamin C to function properly.

There are many camu camu products to choose from (see the consumer guide in chapter 7) that are reasonably priced, and many are now organic products. With more people trying to reduce GMOs in their diet, camu camu is a great option to achieve optimal vitamin C levels for optimal health without the possible GMOs in synthetic chemical vitamin C supplements.

Remember, camu camu is more than just the vitamin C it contains. In the next chapter, we'll look at the other important natural antioxidant compounds found in camu camu and how all these natural chemicals work together synergistically to fight free radicals, relieve oxidative stress and chronic inflammation, and interrupt the progression of chronic diseases.

CHAPTER 4

The Power of Polyphenols

In addition to a therapeutic level of vitamin C, camu camu is a rich source of natural polyphenol chemicals that include anthocyanins, flavonoids, and phenolic acids. In fact, camu camu delivers almost as many polyphenols as it does vitamin C, so it's an important aspect that adds to the benefits and actions of camu camu far beyond its vitamin C levels. The amount of these polyphenols can vary in camu camu fruit (and all fruits and plants), which will be discussed in this chapter. You'll learn why polyphenols are important and how they contribute to the many documented actions and benefits of camu camu for numerous purposes.

You'll also learn that, of all known plant compounds, polyphenols have repeatedly been shown to be the most powerful for protecting against chronic diseases, including heart disease, clogged arteries, metabolic disorders like type 2 diabetes, dementia, Alzheimer's disease, Parkinson's disease, and other degenerative brain diseases. Because they are the most protective, they are also the most preventative.

What Is a Polyphenol?

We've known about plant polyphenols for quite a few years, and they've been studied extensively. Over 80,000 research studies have been published on polyphenols since the mid-1980s, and research continues today at a fast pace. More than 8,000 different polyphenols have been identified thus far, and we continue to discover new ones, mostly in medicinal plants and novel tropical fruits.

Polyphenols are unique natural plant compounds that can be found in all plants and, typically, almost all parts of the plants—leaves, stems, barks, fruits, fruit peels or skin, seeds, and roots. Every plant contains a unique combination of polyphenols, which is why different plants and fruits, all rich in these substances, can have very different effects on the body.

All living things have inbred survival instincts. It is literally part of the cellular makeup of all species on earth. In highly mobile species like humans and other animals, the main survival instinct and mechanism is "flee, fight, or hide." Even bacteria and virus species have learned to flee or hide from immune cells and chemical agents attacking them, as well as to fight them by mutating or changing their own physical structure to defend against them. With stationary plants rooted to the ground and incapable of physically fleeing from danger, their survival instinct is controlled by wonderfully complex and rich chemical defense mechanisms that have evolved over eons. Plants have either created a chemical defense mechanism against what might harm them, or they have succumbed and become extinct. This is the mechanism the plants use to survive, grow, and flourish as well as to fight the many disease-causing organisms that attack them. Creating and utilizing polyphenols is one of the main mechanisms plants use to survive, grow, and flourish, to fight the many disease-causing organisms that attack them, as well as repair the damage they've caused.

Polyphenols are created in plants as a part of a plant's unique biochemical immune system and antioxidant system. These chemicals reduce free radicals and prevent or repair the damage caused by free radicals that the plants are exposed to. Oxidative damage in plants can be a result of less than perfect growing conditions, soil toxins and heavy metals, too much or too little water, too much or too little sunlight, and other negative conditions. Polyphenols are also the healing and repairing agents in plants' specialized "immune systems" to overcome and heal damage by insects and browsing animals, and to protect it from various microbes like plant viruses, bacteria, fungi, and mold.

This is why the type and number of polyphenols can vary widely in plants and the same plants can vary in polyphenol levels from one growing season to another. It really all depends on what types of damage and negative growing conditions the plants had to overcome by increasing its polyphenol content. The more stressful conditions, the higher the polyphenol content. It is also for this reason that wild-harvested plants usually have more polyphenols than cultivated plants. Growers of cultivated plants, like fruits and vegetables and even medicinal plants, control stress factors to their crops to increase harvesting yields . . . from proper irrigation, added soil nutrients, insect control, and even protection from intense sunlight. Controlling these factors will result in the plant needing to produce less stress-reducing and healing polyphenols.

These aspects also explain why tropical fruits like camu camu usually have higher amounts and more diversity in their polyphenol content than cultivated fruits in the United States or Europe. The growing conditions in the tropics are just more intense and stressful. High humidity (which promotes more mold and fungi), intense heat and sunlight, and periods of monsoon-like rains followed by dry periods in the typical rainy-dry seasons of the tropics all contribute to the need of tropical plants to increase polyphenol production to protect themselves. And let's not forget about the bugs! Without a cold season to kill off crawling bugs as well as bacteria, viruses, and fungi, the diversity of pests that tropical plants are exposed to are *much* higher in the tropics than in temperate climates. When botanists say a particular plant has "adapted" to grow in the tropics, this adaptation is usually all about the plant's having increased its natural polyphenol production enough to survive in these more extreme growing conditions.

The consumption of exotic tropical fruits has gained in popularity in both domestic and international markets due to the growing recognition of their much higher nutritional and health-promoting effects. Fruit juices and dried fruit powders from camu, camu, acerola, acai, guava, graviola, maqui berry, passionfruit, mango, and others are showing up in many functional foods and beverages as well as in dietary supplements in the natural products industry. And it's usually all about the powerful and high number of polyphenols these tropical fruits provide.

How Polyphenols Are Unique

The main feature that makes a polyphenol a polyphenol is its unique molecular structure, which usually makes them easy to identify. The manner in which the compound is put together molecularly facilitates a polyphenol to easily attach to and bond to other molecules and chemicals, oftentimes creating brand-new compounds. This unique molecular structure also makes polyphenols especially attracted to enzyme chemicals. However, rather than creating a new compound, they often bond to the enzyme and then disable the enzyme from performing its job, making them effective enzyme inhibitors.

For example, one of the reasons most polyphenols have antioxidant actions is that polyphenols are capable of binding with and interfering with two enzymes that are required in the complicated biochemical chain of events that creates a free radical, and especially ROS free radicals. Another good example is this: Some polyphenols are reported with weight loss or blood sugar–lowering actions because those polyphenols bond to and disable the digestive enzymes we produce during digestion that break down sugars and starches in our meals. If these enzymes don't do their job, then the sugar and starches (and their calories) are not broken down and absorbed (raising blood sugar levels and promoting weight gain), and they are eliminated undigested. Not all polyphenols can provide this benefit/action, but some can.

Polyphenols can bind with almost any type of compound—with sugars, with other plant chemicals, and even with each other. These types of new compounds are usually called derivatives or isomers of the chemical a polyphenol connected with. For example, there are two very common natural acids found in many fruits, vegetables, and medicinal plants called caffeic acid and quinic acid. When these two chemicals bind with one another, they create new chemicals that are basically combinations or bonds between these two plant chemicals. These bonds form isomers. One very well-known isomer of caffeic and quinic acids is chlorogenic acid (CGA). So far, more than 71 different CGA compounds have been reported and are widely distributed in plants. These various compounds are just slightly different derivatives of caffeic acid bonding with quinic acid, but actions, benefits, and absorption of these derivatives can be very different.

The binding action of polyphenols can happen inside plants to make more healing and antioxidant chemicals when the plant needs them, and these bonds can happen and new chemicals are formed inside our bodies during digestion. These types of chemicals are called metabolites—a product of metabolism. Unbelievably, while scientists have confirmed there are more than 8,000 unique polyphenols, they estimate that between 100,000 and 200,000 metabolites of polyphenols are created in plants, animals, humans, and even microbes like bacteria. This makes it harder for scientists to study since digestive processes are so unique, very difficult to create inside a test tube, are often different in laboratory animals than in humans, and are even different among individual humans. To make matters more complicated, some of these polyphenols are not easily digested, and they make it to the colon where we each have our own unique ratio of thousands of gut bacteria species that make up our gut microbiome. Landmark research over the last five years has shown that polyphenols interacting with bacteria in the gut microbiome make a whole host of new chemicals that contribute to many physiological functions. From chemicals that control our appetite, insulin sensitivity, fat storage, fat burning, and inflammation levels to the manufacture of neurotransmitters we need for mood, brain function, and much more, polyphenols are now thought to be the best way to modulate our gut bacteria to promote health.

We will probably never know the total effect polyphenols and their many isomers, derivatives, and metabolites have on promoting heath and treating diseases, but scientists agree, it's a fascinating subject that promotes rigorous ongoing research on these important natural compounds.

The Main Actions of Polyphenols

While every natural plant chemical can have unique actions and benefits, polyphenol compounds generally share some common properties and actions. These shared actions are detailed next.

Antioxidant Actions

Almost without exception, polyphenols are widely documented as strong antioxidants. Not only can they quench free radicals, but they have cellular-protective effects to protect cells and organs from the damaging oxidation and resulting cellular damage that free radicals cause. Utilizing their binding actions with enzymes, polyphenols interfere in the chemical chain of events that's required to make a free radical. Some polyphenols can also encourage the production of our own natural antioxidant enzymes to help address free radicals.

The powerful antioxidant nature of polyphenols has been demonstrated repeatedly in research to prevent or treat various diseases and conditions where oxidative stress is a factor in the development or progression of the disease—of which there are many. In addition, polyphenols are typically called "chain-breaking" antioxidants and are very important to add to vitamin antioxidants like vitamin C. When vitamin C lends an electron to a free radical, it becomes a pro-oxidant itself, and with two missing electrons, it can actually become a free radical, causing cellular damage until it is quenched by another antioxidant. When polyphenols lend electrons, they remain fairly stable and so prevent the initiation of further radical reactions. Polyphenols can also lend electrons to unstable vitamin C intermediates and "break the chain" reaction of vitamins turning from antioxidants to pro-oxidants to free radicals. In many studies, the antioxidant actions of polyphenols are documented to be four to five times more effective at relieving oxidative stress than the typical vitamin antioxidants (vitamins C, A, and E) which mainly lend electrons to free radicals.

Anti-inflammatory Actions

The majority of polyphenols have shown some sort of anti-inflammatory action. Oftentimes inflammation is relieved or reduced simply by reducing free radicals and their damaging effects. You'll learn how oxidative stress causes chronic inflammation in the next chapter. Some polyphenols reduce inflammation by interfering in the biochemical chain of events our immune system uses to cause inflammation. This results in changes in the biochemical process where fewer pro-inflammatory chemicals are produced by the immune system and overall inflammation is reduced. This is considered an immune-regulating or immune-modulation action even though the end result is less inflammation. Again, more on inflammation in general follows in the next chapter.

Antimicrobial Actions

Many polyphenols have been shown to effectively kill bacteria, viruses, and fungi in humans, just as they do in plants. This can make some polyphenols and polyphenol-rich foods natural antimicrobial agents to aid in treating infections. These antimicrobial actions are also playing a role in the friendly bacteria (and not so friendly bacteria) in our gut microbiome. The antibacterial actions of polyphenols can kill off certain types of gut bacteria, yet paradoxically, other friendly bacteria are immune and use polyphenols as a food source (prebiotic) to increase in strength and numbers. Most of the gut microbiome research with polyphenols indicate they can modulate the bacterial species in a manner to treat obesity, help maintain a healthy weight more easily, reduce intestinal inflammation, and treat or prevent chronic bowel diseases such as irritable bowel syndrome and inflammatory bowel diseases.

Modulates Cholesterol

The majority of polyphenols play a beneficial role in the biochemical processes of how the human body processes fat in the diet. This benefit is largely attributed to the antioxidant action of polyphenols and preventing the changes in the biochemical process that occur from the actions of free radicals. The effects of free radicals can result in oxidized fat cells, causing deregulated cholesterol and triglyceride levels, the promotion of clogged arteries, and heart and vein damage, leading to high blood pressure and heart diseases. A classification of antioxidants called anthocyanins are the strongest among the polyphenols that benefit the heart and cholesterol levels.

Modulates Blood Sugar Levels

Polyphenols from different plant-based sources, including those found in camu-camu have been shown to influence glucose metabolism in several ways. These include as inhibition of starch digestion and sugar absorption in the intestine, stimulation of insulin secretion from the pancreatic β-cells, modulation of glucose release from the liver, activation of insulin receptors and glucose uptake in insulin-sensitive tissues, and modulation of liver glucose output. Many polyphenol-rich plants and foods are promoted as antidiabetic or beneficial for the treatment or prevention type 2 diabetes for these reasons. More information concerning camu camu's polyphenols which have the ability to modulate blood sugar levels is found in chapter 6.

Anti-Aging Actions

A significant number of polyphenols have shown the ability to prolong the lifespan of laboratory animals in new anti-aging research. Again, free radicals are implicated in the overall aging process in both humans and animals. They can accumulate over the years in our bodies, resulting in state of chronic oxidative stress at old age. This affects not only our skin but also many internal cells, organs, and biochemical processes.

Inside most of our cells are organelles called mitochondria, and they play an integral role in biochemical processes going on inside our cells. Mitochondria, which are often called the powerhouses of cells, act like miniature factories, converting the food we eat into usable energy in the form of a chemical called adenosine triphosphate (ATP). ATP provides energy to fuel a myriad of cellular processes. If there is a biochemical process going on inside a cell, it is typically going on in the mitochondria.

Mitochondria are actually a significant generator of free radicals because free radicals are a byproduct of creating ATP. Each of our cells contain a little bit of vitamin C and antioxidant enzymes, and their role is to help deactivate these mitochondrial-produced free radicals. However, mitochondria can also be a target of free radical damage if our natural antioxidant system isn't doing its job effectively, leading to mitochondrial dysfunction. Research now reports that mitochondrial dysfunction is one of the root causes of aging, and it helps create a state of chronic oxidative stress in the elderly. As our cells age, mitochondria lose their ability to provide cellular energy efficiently and release more free radicals, including ROS, that harm cells.

Significant research on polyphenols has reported that these naturally strong and cellular-protective antioxidant compounds can treat and relieve mitochondrial dysfunction. Restoring mitochondrial function basically renews the cell and allows it to function like it did when it was much younger. This is one method by which polyphenols can deliver an anti-aging effect and why they can prolong life in animal studies. However, another significant factor in aging is the accumulation and damage of other free- radical–like substances called advanced glycation end products (AGEs). AGEs also accumulate in our bodies, cells, and organs as we age, and are considered to be the hallmark of cellular aging. The levels of AGEs in our bodies are now thought to directly relate to how well or poorly we age, as well as which age-related chronic diseases we are at risk for.

Again, the research on these powerful polyphenols are revealing that maybe the best natural compounds on the planet that are capable of reducing AGEs and protecting cells and biochemical processes from their damaging effects are polyphenols. Thousands of studies on polyphenols (including those found in camu camu) report the anti-aging benefits these effective compounds can provide. See chapter 6 for more information on AGEs and problems they cause and why camu camu was reported in research to provide these AGE-inhibiting and anti-aging benefits.

The Polyphenols in Camu Camu

As discussed in this chapter, polyphenol amounts in fruits and plants can vary depending on growing conditions.

You'll also learn in chapter 7, the consumer guide section of this book, that polyphenol amounts can also vary based on harvesting and processing methods. Typically, polyphenol contents in camu camu are shown to range from 110 to 120 milligrams in just one gram (1,000 mg) of dried camu camu fruit powder. This is substantially higher than one can obtain from the regular fruits and vegetables in a normal diet, even those considered to be good sources of polyphenols.

For example, broccoli is considered a high-polyphenol vegetable that is being promoted as a healthy food to consume in the diet and also sold as a functional food in various dried vegetable powder supplements. The polyphenol content of a dried broccoli vegetable powder has shown to contain about 8 milligrams of polyphenols per gram of dried broccoli which far less than camu camu's 110 milligrams. And to get the equivalent polyphenols by just adding fresh broccoli to your diet, several pounds daily would need to be consumed to equal just one gram of dried camu camu powder. Also keep in mind, that broccoli would need to be eaten raw, since the polyphenols in broccoli (and other nutrients like vitamin C) leach out when it's cooked in boiling water.

To date, camu camu has been reported to contain 53 different powerful polyphenols. Since these natural compounds can bind to other chemicals during digestion and when the plants call on them for defensive actions, the total number of polyphenol compounds and the metabolites they create when we consume camu camu can be much greater. The most significant (by volume) comes from a polyphenol called ellagic acid. This phenolic acid and at least eight of its discovered derivatives make up almost half of camu camu's polyphenol content. Ellagic acid has been the subject of more than 4,000 studies over the years, and this beneficial polyphenol compound has been documented with antioxidant, anti-obesity, anti-inflammatory, anticancer, antimicrobial, enzyme-inhibitor, antidiabetic, and neuro-, cardio-, and liver-protector actions, among others. Some of camu camu's researched actions are attributed to this phenolic acid; however, it is well documented that all of camu camu's many polyphenols are working together synergistically, thereby contributing to the net effect of camu camu's many benefits and actions. Camu camu also provides a good supply of catechin and cyanidin polyphenols, which have also been documented with many derivatives and metabolites in both the fruit as well as in animals and human who consume the fruit.

The polyphenols camu camu provides include castalagin, catechin and its derivatives, chlorogenic acid, cyanidin and its derivatives, delphinidin and its derivatives, ellagic acid and its derivatives, ellagitannins, epicatechins, epigallocatechins, ferulic acid, gallic acid and its gallotannin derivatives, kaempferol derivatives, luteolin, malvidin and its derivatives, myricetin and its derivatives, naringenin, pelargonidin and its derivatives, peonidin, petunidin, rutin, quercetin and its derivatives, quercitrin and isoquercitrin, and syringic acid.

Different Polyphenols Means Different Actions

While all plants contain polyphenols, each plant has its own unique blend of these natural compounds that usually results in what each plant's overall benefits are. With more than 8,000 polyphenols to choose from in nature, the differences between the health benefits of different plants can be the specific polyphenols a plant contains. The next clue is to look at the actions of each polyphenol and their effective dosages to achieve a benefit. Some polyphenols work at extremely low dosages of just a microgram or two to derive a benefit, and others need much higher amounts. Even common spices like cinnamon and cloves, culinary herbs like oregano and thyme, and many medicinal plants are significant sources of beneficial polyphenols, which can be greater than those found in vegetables. And, as previously discussed, tropical fruits like camu camu deliver a much greater amount of polyphenols than standard cultivated fruits and vegetables.

Another interesting factor concerning polyphenols is their ability to target specific kinds of cells, enzymes, molecules, and organs. Some polyphenols have an affinity to target enzymes that result in weight loss, others target cells in the cardiovascular system, and still others target other types of cells, enzymes, or organs like the brain, endocrine system, liver, skin, etc. For example, the polyphenol profile of camu camu is *much* different from the polyphenol profile of broccoli. Camu camu contains anthocyanins (and a significant amount of them), while broccoli contains little to none of this specific type of polyphenol (unless you're eating purple broccoli). Anthocyanins have an affinity to benefit cells, organs, and enzymes in the cardiovascular system and will deliver those benefits much better than other polyphenols found in broccoli. For this reason, you'll see many more anthocyanin-rich purple, blue, and red fruits and vegetables being marketed as "heart-healthy" supplements than many other green vegetables or yellow fruits.

All polyphenols can fight free radicals almost equally, but the affinity to specific cell types usually affects where in the body these polyphenols migrate to and relieve and repair cellular oxidation and damage caused by free radicals. Oftentimes, the best way to determine these affinities is by testing the polyphenol-rich whole plant in animals and humans. *In vitro* testing just confirms the initial antioxidant ability of a plant to quench free radical inside a test tube. Scientists introduce the plant to known pro-oxidant free radical molecules in a test tube and measure how much of the plant substance was required to disable and neutralize the free radicals. While this confirms a plant's antioxidant ability, it has little to do with what actually happens inside the body (*in vivo*) and how these compounds get digested and where they go to interact with free radicals inside us.

For that reason, chapter 6 is all about the animal and human research that has been conducted on camu camu. The research confirms where camu camu's polyphenols are going and which cells and organs are achieving a reduction of free radicals and their damaging effects to provide health benefits. This kind of research is much more important and revealing than the many *in vitro* studies that have been conducted to confirm that camu camu is an effective antioxidant.

The Takeaway

Hopefully what you've learned in this chapter is that polyphenols are important compounds that should be an essential component in your daily diet. This chapter has also revealed why vitamin C–rich *and* polyphenol-rich supplements like camu camu are much ymore beneficial than a single-chemical, synthetic vitamin C supplement. I've always said that nature is a much better chemist than we, as mere mortals, could ever be. Most all plants that have significant levels of vitamin C also have significant levels of polyphenols, almost without exception. What we learned from the previous chapter is that while vitamin C is crucial to our built-in antioxidant system and very good at lending electrons to free radicals, you need other chain-breaking antioxidants like polyphenols to interrupt the normal process of vitamin C turning into first a pro-oxidant and then a free radical after losing its electron(s) to other free radicals.

So nature included high polyphenols in high-vitamin C plants, and so should we! If you're not getting enough vitamin C in your diet, you're probably not getting enough polyphenols either. Taking high dosages of synthetic vitamin C with a low-polyphenol diet may have the opposite effect and actually increase free radical production and oxidative stress instead of relieving it.

Before we review the actual research on camu camu, the next chapter will explain how unrelieved high free radicals in our bodies promote diseases and conditions that could be completely avoided. This information will tell you why camu camu provides a significant benefit in preventing diseases, as confirmed through research on this tropical superfruit. It will also explain why poor diets and our typical "Western diet" is lacking in adequate polyphenols and can be full of free radical–producing foods. The changes in our average diet over the last 30 or so years has significantly increased the amount of preventable chronic diseases we are experiencing in our society as a whole. From obesity and cholesterol problems to heart and brain diseases and many more, in addition to the dwindling amount of fresh, raw, polyphenol-rich, and nutrient-rich fruits, vegetables, and whole grains in our diets, there's been a significant toll on our health.

CHAPTER 5

How Camu Camu
Prevents Disease

A merica is in the middle of a healthcare crisis. Not only are healthcare and insurance costs rising each year, the quickly rising number of people facing chronic diseases are packing doctors' offices at a rapid pace. That polyphenols and natural antioxidants like vitamin C can make a huge impact on preventing diseases almost sounds too simple and too good to be true. However, if you look at the radical changes that have taken place in our diet and lifestyles and relate that to the rise of chronic disease, it's not so hard to understand.

Over the last 50 years, the average American diet has changed significantly. If one takes a step back and looks at the overall broad changes, the most significant factor seen is that our diets consist of food that's lacking in essential vitamins, minerals, and antioxidant polyphenols and includes far too many types of food that promote free radical production and/or harm our built-in natural antioxidant system. The end result has our protective antioxidant system in a state a crisis, which has contributed to the significant rise in chronic diseases we're faced with today. This chapter will discuss how our diet has changed our antioxidant levels and explain how you can avoid the most common chronic and age-related diseases to promote a longer and heathier life with an antioxidant-rich diet or antioxidant-rich supplements like camu camu.

The Western Diet

The average Western diet is low in polyphenols, and the so-called advancements we've made in how we process food over the years seems to be all about removing polyphenols from the food we eat. For example, the largest supply of polyphenols in grains are in the coating of the grain seeds. We went from eating lots of healthy polyphenol-rich whole grains to consuming processed white flour and white rice with the seed coating removed. That is how whole wheat is processed into white flour—they remove the darker-colored polyphenol-rich coating of the seed. This has lowered our polyphenol intake levels significantly.

Starches

The Western diet contains lots of starchy processed foods using white flour. Cakes, cookies, white bread, starchy sweet cereals . . . we are consuming way too many calories from starches in our diet that are lacking in any polyphenols. It isn't surprising that the main vegetable eaten in the Western diet is starchy potatoes. The popularity of french fries isn't going away anytime soon! Most of the polyphenols in potatoes are in the skin, which is usually removed during processing. The high starch in the Western diet increases overall calories of average meals, and when you combine that with less physical exercise in our more sedentary lifestyles, it ends up as one of the causes of weight gain and obesity. But as you'll learn soon, just having less polyphenols in your diet or having chronic oxidative stress is another important cause of weight gain and obesity in the rapidly expanding world population—expanding in weight faster than in population numbers.

Fats

Instead of natural butter and animal fat (lard) comprising most of the fat we used to consume, hydrogenated vegetable oils and margarines replaced them. Butter is a source of polyphenols and essential fat-soluble vitamin antioxidants, as well as important essential fatty acids that act as antioxidants and anti-inflammatory agents. Even animal fats contain polyphenols and beneficial fatty acids.

Additionally, infusing today's manufactured fats and oils with hydrogen to extend their shelf-life promotes more reactive oxygen species (ROS) free radicals to form as our bodies try to digest them. Frying foods repeatedly in the same hydrogenated vegetable oil (think fast-food french fries and fried chicken) actually creates free radicals in the oil, so eating these types of fried food raises our free radical levels because we are actually consuming more free radicals.

So instead of our dietary fats providing natural anti-oxidants to fight free radicals, the fats we are consuming today contain free radicals and/or promote the creation of free radicals. In fact, it is the polyphenol profile of olive oil that makes this oil a great "healthy oil"—olive oil is full of polyphenols. It's also why butter is making a comeback as being a "healthy fat" again and why you should consider adding butter and olive oil to your diet to replace some of the margarine and hydrogenated oils you currently consume. See the section "Cardiovascular Diseases" later in this chapter to learn how the antioxidant nature of these natural saturated fats can help prevent heart diseases rather than increase heart risks due to higher saturated-fat consumption.

Sugars

White sugar and high-fructose corn syrup (HFCS) have replaced the brown sugar, honey, molasses, and other natural sugars we used to consume. The one thing in common among the natural sugars we no longer eat regularly is their polyphenol content. Processing sugarcane or beets into white sugar removes all the polyphenols, which usually taste bitter. The actual sugarcane and beet plants are full of polyphenols; the processed white sugar from these plants has none.

More alarming, scientists now report that consuming HCFS can slow the production and action of our natural enzyme antioxidants, which we need to keep free radicals in check. You'd be amazed at how quickly your free radical levels would decrease if you just eliminated the sodas and fruit juices with HFCS from your diet. When I read this new research, I wondered whether high-HFCS foods should bear a warning label just like cigarettes do. Both generate an unhealthy level of free radicals with inevitable health issues. While consuming too much of any kind of sugar has established negative health effects, the high level of white sugar and HFCS is one of the main negative effects in the Western diet that increases our risks of developing chronic diseases.

Fruits and Vegetables

The Western diet is also very low in raw fruits and vegetables. As a society, we are consuming way too much processed and fast foods in our busy lives, and these types of meals are severely lacking in fruits and vegetables. Fresh fruits and vegetables are supposed to be the main source of polyphenols in our diet. Researchers looking at this aspect of diet and nutrition in the modern diet reported that the main source of polyphenols in the Western diet now comes from coffee and chocolate. Polyphenols from vegetables in the diet came in dead last. Even drinking wine (which contains polyphenols) was higher than vegetables in their analyses. This is mostly because we just aren't eating the daily recommendation of nine servings of fruits and vegetables a day—and usually far less than that. And if one or more of those servings in our diet is a fruit juice loaded with HFCS, it doesn't really count since it will do more harm than good for our antioxidant system!

While coffee and chocolate do contain a significant amount of polyphenols (the polyphenol profile is similar in both sources), those who consume them are still missing many other important beneficial polyphenols from other foods sources. And let's face it, fruits and vegetables are also an important and main source of the vitamins and minerals in our diets that we need to be healthy—chocolate and coffee are pretty lacking in that department. In fact, the researchers studying the natural antioxidants in modern diets noted that when you look at all antioxidants consumed in modern diets, those coming from vitamin-type antioxidants (vitamins A, C, and E) represented less than 10 percent of the total natural antioxidants consumed. We simply cannot rely on just coffee and chocolate (or wine) alone for the polyphenols we need—not if we want to stay healthy.

The Net Results of Poor Diets

Basically, the hallmark of a Western diet is the lack of essential nutrients we need, including natural vitamins and polyphenols that keep our antioxidant system humming along and doing its job of keeping free radicals in check. Havoc ensues when our antioxidant system falters or we're consuming too many empty calories from foods lacking in these nutrients and which promote more free radicals instead.

Before we discuss what damage and diseases oxidative stress causes, you need to know about chronic inflammation. You may be surprised to learn that one of the main deregulations and effects that free radicals cause is raising the level of inflammation in our bodies. Oxidative stress and chronic inflammation go hand in hand and have surfaced as the "root of all evil" when it comes to chronic diseases. Free radicals and inflammation are uniquely intertwined since inflammation promotes the creation of free radicals and free radicals promote inflammation—they are reacting together in a self-perpetuating cycle that leads to the development of multiple diseases.

The Inflammation Connection

Inflammation seems to be the new buzzword in the health industry, in both conventional and natural health circles—as well it should be. Tens of thousands of researchers and scientists around the world have documented the major role that inflammation plays in health and disease, and their discoveries are staggering. We now know that inflammation can be a cause of or a contributing factor to a wide range of disorders, including almost every chronic disease. There are even new anti-inflammatory diet and recipe books being published these days, teaching readers how they can modify their diets to reduce inflammation. And, if you read them, most promote excluding foods that promote the generation of free radicals (the wrong kinds of fats and sugars) and adding lots of polyphenol-rich fruits and vegetables.

Some books and researchers talk about the connection between free radicals and chronic inflammation, and some only focus on the inflammation factor. However, what everyone should be learning is that the main cause of chronic inflammation is the negative effect of too many free radicals damaging cells in many parts of the body. Free radical damage causes inflammation. Taking antioxidants instead of anti-inflammatories can well treat the underlying causes of chronic inflammation in addition to the diseases they cause instead of just treating the inflammatory symptoms. Once you get your antioxidant system healthy and humming along as well as reduce your free radical load, you don't need to take anti-inflammatories to just treat symptoms. As a naturopath, I've long looked for root causes of diseases instead of relying on mainstream approaches of focusing and treating symptoms instead.

When most people think of inflammation, they think of the body's temporary response to injury and infection—a response that can be painful but is an essential part of the body's healing process. Unfortunately, not all inflammation is beneficial to the body. To understand why, we have to look at the difference between acute and chronic inflammation and how free radicals cause chronic inflammation.

Acute Inflammation

Acute inflammation is where our immune system shines. When we suffer an injury, such as a sprained ankle, chemical messengers known as cytokines are released by the damaged tissue and cells at the site of injury. These cytokines act as "emergency signals" that send out more of the body's immune cells, hormones, and nutrients. Blood vessels dilate and blood flow increases so that the healing agents can move quickly into the blood to flood the injured area. This inflammatory response is what causes the ankle to turn red and become swollen. As the healing agents go to work, the ankle is repaired, and the inflammation gradually subsides.

When you get a cut or wound, the same thing happens. Special white blood cells (known as natural killer cells) along with clotting and scabbing nutrients rush to the area to prevent infection, stop the bleeding, and form a scab. Again, the body's response causes redness and inflammation around the wound, but it is a sign that your immune system is at work protecting you from infection and healing the injury. Without this natural inflammatory response, wounds would fester and infections would abound.

Chronic Inflammation

Long-term, or chronic, inflammation is different from acute inflammation, and it's where our immune system and our natural inflammatory processes can cause problems. Chronic inflammation is also called persistent, low-grade inflammation because it can produce a steady, low level of inflammation throughout the body. This condition has been proven to contribute to many diseases, and research suggests it may cause some common chronic diseases such as diabetes, heart diseases, and even aging. Low levels of inflammation can be triggered by a perceived internal threat—just as an injury triggers acute inflammation—even when there isn't a disease to fight or an injury to heal. This can activate the body's natural immune response, and inflammation is the result.

Free Radicals: The Leading Cause of Chronic Inflammation

The cellular damage caused by free radicals is the main perceived threat in our bodies that activates the immune system to cause inflammation. When healthy cells become damaged or begin dying from free radical damage, the body triggers the immune system to start the inflammatory process in an effort to repair or remove the cells. Because free radicals are distributed throughout the body, and the cellular damage is occurring cell by cell wherever a free radical interacts with a healthy cell, the inflammatory response spreads throughout the body. The cell-by-cell damage is smaller than damage caused by injury or infection, so the inflammation response is much smaller. This results in low levels of chronic inflammation throughout the body as the immune system tries to do its job of cleaning up or repairing free radical–damaged cells.

Unfortunately, when an imbalance occurs between the production of free radicals and the ability of the body to counteract these substances' negative effects, a negative feedback loop can be generated. In some cells and systems in the body, oxidative stress causes inflammation, and the inflammation can trigger the generation of even more free radicals. Then these additional free radicals create more oxidative stress, which causes more inflammation—a vicious cycle is created, and everything become chronic. It is important to understand that this process may have a detrimental effect on every one of our cells and in many of our complicated internal biochemical processes in different organs. This negative cycle can continue silently, usually without any outward symptoms or signs, causing us significant risks of developing chronic disease without even knowing.

While free radical damage can be the biggest cause of chronic inflammation, it's certainly not the only cause. But that's where polyphenol antioxidants can play a huge role and a greater one than vitamin antioxidants and our own natural enzyme antioxidants can. Most all polyphenols have antioxidant *and* anti-inflammatory actions. Polyphenols work in several ways to reduce and relieve inflammation, not just through reducing free radicals. Whether a problem is created by oxidative stress or chronic inflammation, polyphenols can be effective—if you pick the plants that have the right polyphenol combinations and profiles.

Prevent Diseases Caused by Oxidative Stress and Chronic Inflammation

Tens of thousands of research studies have been published on chronic inflammation and oxidative stress and the roles they play in numerous diseases. We now know that inflammation and oxidative stress can be a cause or a contributing factor to a wide range of diseases, including almost every chronic disease. From heart diseases, diabetes, Alzheimer's disease, and cancer to high cholesterol levels, autoimmune diseases, and even obesity—chronic inflammation and oxidative stress are playing significant roles. Many of these studies reveal that when you reduce oxidative stress and chronic inflammation it has a beneficial impact on these conditions. Better yet, if you manage your levels of oxidative stress and chronic inflammation levels with polyphenol antioxidants, you can avoid developing these many conditions. Polyphenol compounds with antioxidant and anti-inflammatory actions, including those found in camu-camu, have surfaced in all this research as the most important natural plant compounds available to us that have the ability to help prevent these diseases.

Obesity

New research indicates that obesity is actually a chronic inflammatory disease, and the fatty tissues of overweight individuals are inflamed and suffering from oxidative stress and immune cell damage. When fat cells and fatty tissues are damaged by inflammation and oxidative stress, they do not produce enough of certain natural metabolic chemicals that are required to reduce inflammation, store and burn fats, maintain insulin sensitivity, and support a healthy weight.

Scientists have now discovered more than 80 adipokines that are secreted by fat cells, many of which have known metabolic actions. Research has increased significantly on these natural fat-produced substances and their roles in obesity, diabetes, heart diseases, and other disorders since 2010. New knowledge about these substances and their roles have encouraged the development of new drugs targeting this metabolic system in the treatment of obesity, metabolic diseases, and heart conditions.

Since our fatty tissues and fat cells expand as we gain weight, all these fat-secreted deregulations and resulting inflammation and oxidative stress increases as our fat increases. You don't have to be obese either; just gaining some extra weight can start the process and head you down the road to deregulations. These deregulations make it much harder to lose weight, and some can make it virtually impossible to lose weight. Adipokines also help regulate functions in the heart and how we process sugar and insulin. Obesity-caused adipokine deregulations are now the main link of why obesity significantly increases our risks of developing type 2 diabetes and cardiovascular disease.

We once believed that many of us gained weight as we aged mostly because of reduced activity levels. New research is reporting that the accumulation of free radicals and advanced glycation end products (AGEs) as we age may be the cause of deregulations that promotes weight gain and makes it harder to maintain a healthy weight.

Plants that contain strong antioxidant compounds, including camu camu, have been reported in many studies to treat obesity and promote weight loss by reducing free radicals and lowering oxidative stress and chronic inflammation, which repair the deregulations that occur in our fat-produced metabolic adipokines.

A significant amount of research has been conducted in humans and animals on many different polyphenols that report weight-loss benefits and actions. The main mechanisms of actions reported is the reduction of oxidative stress, AGEs, and chronic inflammation, in addition to some polyphenols' ability to lower the calories in foods by blocking digestive enzymes that break down fats, sugars, and starches.

Research on camu camu reports an anti-obesity action as described here, and it will be discussed in the next chapter.

Cardiovascular Diseases

Adipokines produced in our fat cells control how we regulate our blood pressure and fluid balance, create new blood vessels, and how well our hearts contract to regulate blood flow. The direct deregulations of adipokines in fat cells created by obesity is now considered a main reason that, when we gain too much weight, we are at greater risk for developing heart problems.

In addition to fat deregulations, free radicals are particularly damaging to the cells in the heart and cardiovascular system because they are actually circulating in our bloodstream and are in constant contact. Thousands of studies report the mechanisms by which free radicals and the oxidative damage and inflammation they cause can contribute to the development of clogged arteries, high blood pressure, peripheral vascular disease, coronary artery disease, cardiomyopathy, heart failure, and cardiac arrhythmias.

Free radical damage is also the main reason people who smoke cigarettes have *much* higher risks for developing cardiovascular diseases. Cigarette smoke actually contains free radicals, and the chemical reactions smoke creates in the lungs generates significantly more free radicals. Chemicals used in e-cigarettes and vaping solutions are poorly studied for possible free radicals they might produce in the lungs. The recent reports of lung inflammation and lung cell death (the hallmark of free radical damage) doesn't bode well for the safety of these poorly studied chemicals going into your lungs. If you stop smoking, free radical production in your body will drop dramatically and you'll reduce the risk of free radical damage to your heart and cardiovascular system to prevent heart diseases.

Polyphenol antioxidants, including those found in camu camu, are the subject of a substantial body of research documenting their actions and benefits to the cardiovascular system and their ability to prevent heart diseases. Many human, animal, and *in vitro* studies report that polyphenols exert beneficial effects on the vascular system via the increase of antioxidant defenses and reduction of oxidative stress. These beneficial effects include lowering blood pressure, improving endothelial function, inhibiting platelet aggregation (which reduces blot clots), reducing low-density lipoprotein (LDL) cholesterol oxidation (which clogs arteries), and relieving chronic inflammation by reducing inflammatory responses. The link between polyphenol consumption and the reduction of heart disease risk is well established and widely accepted.

Research on camu camu has been published confirming benefits and actions for the heart and modulating cholesterol. These studies will be reviewed in the next chapter.

Diabetes and Metabolic Diseases

Type 2 diabetes is also categorized as a chronic inflammatory disease that is associated with oxidative stress and insulin resistance. The increased production of reactive oxygen species (ROS) or a reduced capacity of the ROS-scavenging antioxidants can lead to abnormal changes in intracellular signaling and result in chronic inflammation and insulin resistance. Prevention of ROS-induced oxidative stress and inflammation can be an important therapeutic strategy to prevent the onset of type 2 diabetes and well as diabetic complications and co-occurring diseases.

New research also reveals that fat cell–produced adipokines play important roles in glucose metabolism and insulin resistance. It is established through human research that adipokines are deregulated in people with diabetes, and these deregulations are one of the underlying reasons obesity or just being overweight increases the risk of developing type 2 diabetes. Since many of these adipokine deregulations can be repaired with substances that reduce inflammation and oxidative stress, polyphenols have evolved as natural substances that can treat or prevent diabetes.

The initiation and progression of diabetes can also be linked to higher AGE levels in the body and the cellular damage, generation of additional free radicals, and inflammation these AGEs cause.

A significant body of research represents important advances related to influence of polyphenols and polyphenol-rich diets on preventing and managing type 2 diabetes. This research reveals that the main methods of actions polyphenols utilize to prevent diabetes include protection of pancreatic beta cells against glucose toxicity; anti-inflammatory and antioxidant effects; inhibition of digestive enzymes, which decrease starch conversion and sugar absorption; and inhibition of AGE production. Anthocyanin-type polyphenols have also been reported to exhibit antidiabetic properties by reducing blood glucose and HbA1c levels as well as improve insulin secretion and resistance in human and animal studies.

Research on camu camu's actions and benefits for diabetes and lowering glucose levels have been published over the last several years and will be reviewed in the next chapter.

Neurodegenerative Diseases and Brain Disorders

Neurodegenerative disorders such as dementia, Parkinson's disease, and Alzheimer's disease represent an increasing problem in our aging societies, primarily as there is an increased prevalence of these diseases with age. These and other neurodegenerative disorders appear to be triggered by multifactorial events; however, oxidative stress and inflammation in the brain underlie most all neurodegenerative diseases and disorders. Neurons in the brain are frequent targets of oxidative stress, and the resulting cellular damage can lead to cell death and deregulation of chemical processes in the brain.

Studies looking at dietary factors and brain disorders report that regular dietary intake of polyphenol-rich foods and/or beverages has been associated with 50 percent reduction in the risk of dementia, a preservation of cognitive performance with aging, a delay in the onset of Alzheimer's disease, and a reduction in the risk of developing Parkinson's disease. Some polyphenols (including some anthocyanins found in camu camu) have been reported to reduce the neurodegeneration associated with the accumulation AGEs during normal and abnormal brain aging.

Research also suggests that some polyphenols (particularly anthocyanins) are able to cross the blood-brain barrier; thus, these polyphenol compounds are likely to be candidates for direct neuroprotective and neuromodulatory actions. Polyphenols are considered to be neuroprotective because they provide a defense against many underlying causes of neurodegenerative diseases, namely oxidative stress, neuroinflammation, protein aggregation, metal toxicity, and mitochondrial dysfunction.

There is also a growing interest in the potential of polyphenols to improve memory, learning, and general cognitive ability. Human studies suggest that polyphenols may have a positive impact on memory and depression, and there is a large body of animal behavioral research to suggest that anthocyanin polyphenols are effective at reversing age-related deficits in spatial working memory, in improving object recognition memory, and in modulating inhibitory fear conditioning.

Liver Diseases

The most leading causes of liver diseases are oxidative stress, lipid peroxidation (the oxidation of fats by free radicals), chronic inflammation, and immune response deregulations. Natural polyphenols have attracted increasing attention as potential agents for the prevention and treatment of liver diseases. Their striking capacities in relieving oxidative stress, lipid metabolism, insulin resistance, and inflammation put polyphenols in the spotlight for the therapies of liver diseases as well as for the prevention of liver diseases. Numerous studies on polyphenols and polyphenol-rich medicinal plants report the liver-protecting ability of these substances. Thousands of animal studies report that cellular-protective polyphenols can protect the liver from just about anything scientists give the animals—liver-toxic drugs, toxic doses of aspirin and alcohol, and other substances or diseases like diabetes, which are known to cause liver damage.

Age-Related Eye Diseases

Oxidative stress and inflammation play a critical role in the initiation and progression of age-related eye abnormalities such as cataracts, glaucoma, diabetic retinopathy, macular degeneration, and even the autoimmune eye disease Sjögren's syndrome. Therefore, natural plant chemicals with proven antioxidant and anti-inflammatory activities, such as carotenoids and polyphenols, could be of benefit in preventing and treating these diseases. Several carotenoids, including lutein, and the polyphenols in camu-camu have shown significant preventive and therapeutic benefits against these eye conditions in animal and human research. In addition, camu-camu provides a therapeutic amount of ellagic acid and two of its derivatives that have been documented with effective aldose reductase inhibitor actions. Aldose reductase inhibitors are a class of drugs and natural compounds being studied as a way to prevent eye and nerve damage in people with diabetes.

Summary

When you understand the importance of polyphenols and how they can prevent many diseases, it's not all that difficult to understand why we're in such a health crisis with the significant rise in chronic diseases we're experiencing today. Our diets no longer contain the natural polyphenols that are necessary to support our antioxidant defenses to keep our oxidative stress and inflammation levels within the healthy levels, and illness ensues. More than 50 percent of the American population is overweight with rising levels of chronic inflammation and oxidative stress, 48 percent have some type of cardiovascular disease led by the increasing number of people with hypertension, and more than 100 million American adults are now living with diabetes or prediabetes. Metabolic syndrome, a prediabetes condition that usually leads to diabetes, now affects 30 percent of the U.S. population.

If your diet is much like the standard Western diet, you should be choosing the dietary supplements you need to overcome the deficiencies that are increasing your risks for ill health and disease. Choosing wholefood sources of polyphenol-rich foods to add to your diet is the best strategy, and, second to that, adding wholefood supplements like camu camu that are rich in essential nutrients as well as in significant levels of beneficial polyphenols can help prevent deficiencies that lead to the preventable chronic diseases discussed in this chapter. For that reason alone, consumers should consider getting their daily vitamin C from camu camu rather than from a single-chemical, synthetic vitamin C supplement.

Now that we've reviewed all the information on how the power of polyphenols contribute to the treatment and prevention of many diseases, it's much easier to understand how an exotic tropical fruit like camu camu can live up to the claims that it can help decrease your risk of developing a host of chronic diseases. The next chapter will look at the actual research that has been conducted specifically on camu camu in humans, animals, and test tubes that confirms these benefits and actions.

CHAPTER 6

The Researched Benefits of Camu Camu

If you've gotten this far through this book, you will have learned that keeping free radicals at low and healthy levels is very important to promote overall health and to avoid disease. You'll also have learned that the high amount of vitamin C and significant amount of antioxidant polyphenols delivered in camu camu makes it a perfect choice to keep your free radicals in check and support your in-house antioxidant system to do its important job. The only other thing necessary is to look at the actual research conducted on camu camu that confirms this superfruit's strong antioxidant action and other benefits. This chapter will review the research on camu camu's benefits and actions conducted by researchers around the world.

Camu Camu's Antioxidant Actions

More than 25 studies have been published to date confirming camu camu's antioxidant actions. There are several tests utilized to measure the antioxidant potential of plants and their compounds. In plant research, a test called the DPPH radical scavenging assay is the most extensively used to determine the antioxidant value for plant samples since it's inexpensive, quick, and accurate. This test has been the most accepted model for evaluating the free radical scavenging activity of any new drug. DPPH is a free radical that reacts with plants or compounds able to donate an electron and render it into a stable molecule.

Scientists place the plant or compound sample in a test tube with the DPPH radicals and measure how much of the plant is required to stabilize the free radicals and how long it takes to do so. Interestingly, the standard reference compound most researchers use to compare the plant sample against is vitamin C since it is the best known and most widely researched natural antioxidant compound. This gives camu camu its advantage over all other plant and fruit sources that contain significant polyphenols—the combination of the highest vitamin C of all fruits with the very high polyphenol content camu camu delivers results in this tropical fruit's measuring with the highest free radical–scavenging actions of any superfruit as determined by the DHHP test.

For example, another high-polyphenol tropical fruit that has gained in popularity in the U.S. natural product market that comes from the Brazilian Amazon is açai (*Euterpe oleracea*). Since about 2005, açai has been widely marketed for the polyphenol antioxidant actions it provides for weight loss, memory enhancement, disease prevention, and anti-aging benefits. It is a popular ingredient in many functional foods and beverages in the marketplace today for its antioxidant benefits. However, if you compare the DHHP test results for camu camu with açai's test results, you'll see camu camu wins the free radical–scavenging ability in this test . . . hands down. It took more than eight times the amount of açai to stabilize the same amount of DHHP radicals as camu camu, and camu camu stabilized the free radicals in 10 minutes compared to 120 minutes for açai. When you consider that camu camu delivers much more vitamin C (2,000 milligrams versus 84 milligrams) and more than twice the amount of polyphenols, it's easy to understand why.

Other researchers comparing DHHP-tested antioxidant actions reported that camu camu exceeded the antioxidant actions of green tea, red wine, pomegranate, vitamin C, and vitamin A—all promoted to fight free radicals. For way too many years, consumers believed camu camu was just about its high vitamin C content. Hopefully, growing consumer awareness of camu camu's superior results to fight free radicals will increase the use and demand for this super fruit in the future.

Another test measuring antioxidant actions of natural substances that is growing in popularity is called an ORAC (oxygen radical absorbance capacity) assay. The ORAC assay is different in that the free radical used in the test (called AAPH) is a ROS-generating free radical that is commonly found in the human body. Additionally, AAPH is reactive with both water- and fat-soluble substances, so it can measure total antioxidant potential better than DHHP in plant samples with water- and fat-soluble antioxidant compounds. Usually the standard control used for comparison of antioxidant abilities for this test is fat-soluble vitamin E, rather than water-soluble vitamin C. One Brazilian research group, using the ORAC antioxidant test, reported in 2010 that camu camu was 10 times higher in antioxidant actions than 21 other native Brazilian fruits analyzed.

Another test can be used called a FRAP assay, which measures the ability of a substance to address the oxidation of metals in the body, which is a significant ROS generator. And yet another antioxidant test that's used is called an ABTS assay (also known as Trolox equivalent antioxidant capacity, or TEAC). When antioxidant actions are tested in animals or humans, other tests are performed that measure the actual hydroxyl and superoxide radical levels in the bloodstream, and/or nitric oxide (a reactive nitrogen free radical), and lipid peroxidation (oxidation of fat) levels. When these levels are reduced following the administration of a drug or natural substance, antioxidant actions are confirmed.

A human study was conducted in 2008 in Japan to determine camu camu's antioxidant and anti-inflammatory actions. They recruited 20 male smokers. (Smoking is well known to dramatically increase free radical levels, which promotes chronic inflammation in habitual smokers.) The participants were randomly assigned into two groups. The first group was given 70 milliliters (2.37

ounces) of camu camu fruit juice daily for seven days (which naturally contained 1,050 milligrams of vitamin C per serving). The second group was administered a 1,050-milligram synthetic vitamin C tablet daily for the same seven days. At the end of seven days, they measured oxidative stress levels (numbers of free radicals in the blood and urine) as well as inflammatory markers (the amount of pro-inflammatory chemicals such as interleukins and tumor necrosis factors, as well as C-reactive protein) and compared the two groups' results. Remarkably, all levels of oxidative stress and inflammation were significantly reduced in the camu camu group while there was no change in the vitamin C group. They concluded their study saying: "Our results suggest that camu camu juice may have powerful anti-oxidative and anti-inflammatory properties, compared to vitamin C tablets containing equivalent vitamin C content. These effects may be due to the existence of unknown anti-oxidant substances besides vitamin C or unknown substances modulating *in vivo* vitamin C kinetics in camu camu."

Camu camu has been tested in every assay method known to measure antioxidant actions, and the bottom line is: camu camu has the strongest antioxidant actions and in all test methods. Most researchers in these many studies attribute camu camu's strong antioxidant actions to the synergy of many polyphenols working in concert with vitamin C rather than any one single chemical or compound, including camu camu's high vitamin C content. Several other studies show that the high potassium level in camu camu is probably increasing the vitamin C absorption and uptake at a cellular level, which gives camu camu a further edge over synthetic supplements. Researchers also note that camu camu has considerable amounts of carotenoids, some of which are converted to vitamin A when digested. Vitamin A is one of the main natural vitamin antioxidants our built-in antioxidant system needs to fight free radicals, and this is also playing a role in camu camu's overall antioxidant abilities.

The last significant thing to note in all the antioxidant studies on camu camu is the comparison of antioxidant abilities related to the ripeness of the fruit and the processing or manufacturing of the fruit into products suitable for foods and dietary supplements. Interestingly, research reveals that as camu camu ripens, vitamin C levels decrease and the polyphenols increase. Research also indicates that the contribution to camu camu's antioxidant actions when harvested ripe are about 60 percent due to polyphenols and 40 percent due to the vitamin C. The bottom line in these many studies is that ripe and mostly ripe camu camu fruit has the highest antioxidant actions, and even with the loss of a bit of vitamin C (about 20 percent), ripe camu camu still contains more vitamin C than most other fruits.

Cellular-Protective Antioxidant Actions

As discussed in chapter 2, plants produce polyphenols to prevent damage as well as heal damage in their leaves, barks, and fruits. These same polyphenols are shown to provide protective, healing, and repairing actions when we consume them. They also have much more efficacy in reducing free radical damage since they do much more than just lend electrons to free radicals.

Several animal studies describe camu camu's cellular-protective abilities indicating camu camu can provide protective actions for the brain, liver, kidneys, and skin. The first study was published in 2010 by researchers in Japan. They evaluated the liver-protecting actions of 12 highly nutritious fruit juices, including camu camu.

They fed rats the fruit juices daily for seven days and then administered a liver toxic drug (d-galactosamine) and measured the amount of protection the juices provided against a control group that received the liver toxic drug without any fruit juice. Camu camu provided the highest amount of protection among all the juices and significantly prevented the liver damage that is normally caused by the drug. Four other tropical fruit juices, including another superfruit called acerola, provided damage-suppressing actions, but camu camu was much stronger at preventing liver injury.

In 2015, Brazilian researchers studied the brain-protective actions of camu camu in an experimentally induced neurodegeneration animal model for Alzheimer's disease and Parkinson's disease. Since overall brain aging and degeneration of the brain is strongly associated with oxidative stress and resulting chronic inflammation, it's not too surprising that scientists are looking at this possible use for a strong antioxidant like camu camu. It's also not surprising that this research reported significant brain protection, and that camu camu protected brain cells from toxicity and brain cell death, and reduced oxidative processes in brain cells.

Researchers in Peru published a rat study in 2019 on camu camu's ability to prevent damage to the kidneys. They administered rats various dosages of camu camu fruit juice along with a drug that causes cell death and intense inflammation to the kidneys and renal system of rats (gentamicin). These researchers also reported that camu camu fruit juice provided significant protection and prevented damage to the kidneys, and in a dose-dependent manner (the higher amount of fruit juice, the higher protective actions).

In the same year, researchers in Brazil published a study to determine if camu camu could protect mice from the toxic and mutagenic (cellular DNA damage) of alcohol. They administered camu camu fruit juice along with ethanol to mice and reported the juice reduced the alcohol-mediated DNA damage in all tissues analyzed (blood, liver, kidney, and bone marrow).

Additionally, camu camu's cellular-protective antioxidant action also helps to protect the skin. Two studies were published in 2012 and 2014, which reported that camu camu could be added to cosmetic formulations, since the fruit increases the sun-protection factor against UVB radiation. This particular benefit was attributed to the high levels of vitamin C and phenolic compounds in the fruit and the antioxidant actions it provides to protect the skin.

Camu camu's confirmed strong antioxidant actions which can reduce chronic inflammation and oxidative stress provides protection from chronic diseases and many other benefits as outlined in the previous chapters on the benefits of vitamin C and polyphenol antioxidants. Supporting your built-in antioxidant system to do its job well with the help of camu camu means you're supporting your overall health and wellness. See the reference section for a listing of the antioxidant and cellular-protective research conducted on camu camu discussed in this chapter.

Anti-Inflammatory Actions

As discussed in previous chapters, oxidative stress and inflammation go hand in hand, since free radicals cause inflammation, and inflammation promotes the generation of more free radicals. Most polyphenols, including those found in camu camu, have long been documented with anti-inflammatory actions for this reason—inflammation is reduced when free radicals and the damage they cause are reduced. Plant antioxidants seem to do this much better than vitamin antioxidants like vitamin C. This was certainly noticed in the human study on camu camu previously discussed in camu camu's antioxidant actions. All participants taking camu camu in the study had a reduction in inflammatory markers and pro-inflammatory chemicals produced by the immune system, which was not experienced by participants who took just a vitamin C supplement.

Looking at thousands of polyphenol studies over the last year shows that these beneficial plant compounds seem to modulate the immune system in such a way to interrupt the chain of events going on to promote widespread chronic inflammation and the continuous production of these pro-inflammatory substances the body is producing. While this action is more about immune modulation, the end result is still much less chronic inflammation. For this reason, many natural polyphenols and the plants that produce them have been studied for various autoimmune disorders and inflammatory bowel conditions—usually with good benefits demonstrated. Additionally, one of the pro-inflammatory chemicals routinely produced in the immune system's anti-inflammatory processes is one called tumor necrosis factor alpha. The chronic, or long-term, elevation of this pro-inflammatory compound promotes the initiation of cancer.

In addition to the human study documenting camu camu's anti-inflammatory actions, several animal studies have been published confirming these actions. Japanese researchers published a study in 2011 noting that pretreatment with camu camu actually blunted the initial inflammatory response in mice in chemical-induced inflammation to their paws and continued providing an anti-inflammatory effect four hours later. These researchers suggested this action was due, in part, to a triterpenoid chemical in good supply in camu camu called betulinic acid, which has been well documented with potent anti-inflammatory actions.

However, camu camu's 50 some-odd anti-inflammatory polyphenols were most probably working synergistically with this isolated compound to provide the overall anti-inflammatory benefits. Particularly the ellagitannins and ellagic acid and its derivatives are the subject of anti-inflammatory research in quite a few studies. Camu camu provides a significant and therapeutic amount of ellagic acid. Ellagic acid has demonstrated very strong anti-inflammatory actions and a wide array of benefits for inflammatory diseases and conditions *in vitro* (in test tubes) and *in vivo* (in animals and humans), including arthritis, osteoarthritis, inflammatory bowel conditions, cardiovascular inflammation related to heart diseases, inflammatory brain disorders, inflammation in various organs caused by diabetes, and many others.

Interestingly, because both ellagic and betulinic acids form many metabolites and derivatives in both plants and humans, it enables drug researchers to work with these natural compounds to easily create new derivatives of both compounds to create new patentable drugs. Both compounds have been synthesized by researchers (created in the laboratory without any plant material or the extracted natural organic compound), and several pharmaceutical companies are trying to turn them into new anti-inflammatory drugs for chronic inflammation, as well as other types of drugs (for obesity and heart diseases). Our current supply of anti-inflammatory drugs are specific to acute inflammation rather than chronic inflammation, are not without negative side effects, and these side effects increase if they are used chronically and long term. While new synthesized ellagic acid and betulinic acid drugs may well be on the horizon, we don't need to wait; camu camu provides therapeutic levels of both compounds naturally, as nature made them, and certainly at a much lower cost than expensive new drugs.

Anti-Aging and AGE-Inhibitor Actions

As discussed in previous chapters, aging has been associated with a chronic low-grade inflammatory state as well as increased oxidative stress. It is widely accepted that reactive oxygen species (ROS) in many cells accumulate over our lifespan and lead to a state of chronic oxidative stress at old age. Low-grade inflammation caused by oxidative stress is also now strongly linked to much higher risks of developing age-related memory loss, dementia, and even Alzheimer's disease. Camu camu's strong antioxidant actions to fight free radicals, including ROS, and relieve oxidative stress and chronic inflammation are at the core of camu camu's ability to promote healthy aging.

However, another huge area of anti-aging research over the last 10 years indicates that reducing advanced glycation end products (AGEs) in the body provides anti-aging benefits. AGEs are harmful compounds that are formed when protein or fat combines or bonds improperly with sugar in the bloodstream. This process is called glycation. These improperly bonded compounds can travel throughout the body and cause a host of problems, including chronic inflammation, cellular damage and cell death, and the interruption of cellular signaling. AGEs also encourage the creation of ROS, which generate oxidative stress and more inflammation. In fact, AGEs and ROS are uniquely intertwined. For an AGE to be created inside the body, the protein or the fat that creates the bond has to be oxidized first, usually by ROS. Therefore, having higher ROS levels means having more AGEs. Once an AGE is created, the damage and inflammation it causes results in the formation of more ROS, and a negative cycle is established.

AGEs and the damage they cause are now linked to cellular aging and premature aging inside the body and in various organs. Over a dozen different AGEs have been identified in the human body, and about half are known to accumulate with age in skin cells, affecting collagen production and promoting wrinkling and thinning of the skin. The rest of the AGEs can start accumulating in other organs and in the bloodstream, causing aging and cellular damage in the heart and cardiovascular system, kidneys, liver, and brain, resulting in chronic age-related diseases in these organs.

The link between AGEs and age-related diseases was recognized as early as 2001, when medical researchers at the University of South Carolina reported in the journal *Experimental Gerontology* that "they [AGEs] accumulate to high levels in tissues in age-related chronic diseases, such as atherosclerosis, diabetes, arthritis and neurodegenerative disease. Inhibition of AGE formation in these diseases may limit oxidative and inflammatory damage in tissues, retarding the progression of pathophysiology and improve the quality of life during aging." Recently, measuring AGE levels in individuals over age 60 has been proposed as a possible new blood test to monitor healthy aging and to enable the early detection of age-related diseases.

If we want to age well, or even slow aging, one of the best ways to accomplish that is to effectively manage our AGE levels. Some polyphenols have shown to be effective AGE-inhibitors in many different studies and camu camu contains ten well-known polyphenol compounds with documented AGE-inhibitor actions. The strongest of these, again, is the ellagic acid and several derivatives that are created in plants and which camu camu delivers in therapeutic amounts.

The ellagic acids and ellagitannins found in camu camu have demonstrated potent inhibitory activities on AGE formation in quite a few other anti-aging studies. Second to that are the betulinic acid, cyanidin, and pelargonidin natural derivatives found in camu camu. Many of the studies on these anti-aging compounds in camu camu report that they can interfere with or prevent the formation of AGEs and/or interrupt the cellular signaling or disable the AGE receptor sites to prevent AGE-related cellular damage.

One of the most recent studies on camu camu's anti-aging action was an industry-standard test. Researchers have developed a special mutated species of flat worm (*Caenorhabditis elegans*) that they regularly use for anti-aging research. If a plant or a substance can prolong the short lifespan of this particular worm, it indicates that the substance might also help prolong the life of humans. Usually plants and plant chemicals passing this test are targeted for further anti-aging research to determine their specific actions in this regard.

Researchers in Brazil published a study in 2015 reporting that camu camu increased the lifespan of this special worm by 20 percent. Their study also reported that camu camu elicited a strong protection against amyloid-ß-induced toxicity. This is the small protein linked to brain cell death and the progression of Alzheimer's disease and Parkinson's disease, which was discussed previously in this chapter in the cellular-protective antioxidant actions camu camu provided to the brain.

A collaboration of university researchers from several American and Brazilian universities also published a study in 2015 concerning camu camu's cellular-regenerative abilities. They used a *Planaria* animal model (a different type of flatworm), which is considered a regenerative model to determine the potential of camu camu's actions for cellular protection and rejuvenation. The potential of *Planaria* is based on the fact that entire sections of the worm can fully regrow from amputated sections of the head or lower tail region. Scientists can evaluate if a plant, fruit, or other substance is able to speed up this process to regenerate itself. Camu camu passed the test with researchers reporting that camu camu increased regeneration between 35 and 50 percent (depending on if freeze-dried or spray-dried camu camu was used).

With camu camu's many antioxidant, anti-inflammatory, and AGE-inhibitor compounds, it's not surprising that researchers chose this anti-aging area of study for camu camu. Nor are their results surprising. Camu camu can promote healthy aging through addressing the three main aspects of why and how (and how fast) we age: chronic inflammation, oxidative stress, and rising AGE levels. The disease-prevention abilities of camu camu as described throughout this book can also provide us a higher quality of life as we get older, reduce the amount of prescription drugs we must take to treat age-related chronic diseases, and promote a healthier, happier, and richer lifestyle as we age. See the reference section for a listing of the research discussed in this section.

Anti-Obesity and Antidiabetic Actions

As discussed in previous chapters, obesity is associated with a decrease in antioxidant capacity, higher levels of damaging free radicals, and the resulting chronic inflammation, and many studies have shown beneficial effects of antioxidant supplementation in treating obesity. In addition, the previously discussed AGE-inhibitor and cellular-protective antioxidant abilities of camu camu hold important information for people with diabetes. Diabetes also causes a significant amount of additional ROS and AGEs in numerous ways, which results in chronic inflammation, oxidative stress, and ongoing AGE damage to organs that leads to the development of diabetes-related complications and co-diseases.

Type 2 diabetes and being overweight usually occur simultaneously, and researchers still argue over the "chicken or egg first" aspect of whether obesity causes diabetes or whether diabetes promotes weight gain and obesity. Both are probably right. Regardless, the main contributing factors (besides a poor diet) for the progression of both conditions are high oxidative stress and the chronic inflammation it causes with natural plant polyphenols surfacing in thousands of studies as effective treatments and for prevention purposes.

Several animal studies have been published determining camu camu's benefits in both diabetes and obesity. In addition to the relief of chronic inflammation and oxidative stress positively affecting both conditions, camu camu provides additional actions. As discussed in chapter 4, polyphenols are effective enzyme inhibitors, and this plays a role in both diabetes maintenance and weight loss. When the digestive enzymes we produce to break down sugars and starches (alpha-glucosidase and alpha-amylase) are inhibited, these starchy and sugary foods are not broken down for absorption and are just eliminated through the stools. That also means the calories from these foods aren't absorbed, which lowers the calories in meals to promote weight loss. In addition, this also reduces the amount of sugar that goes into the bloodstream, which is beneficial for diabetes by lowering blood glucose levels after eating a meal.

Camu camu contains nine polyphenols that inhibit alpha-glucosidase and/or alpha-amylase, and the fruit's ability to block these enzymes has been confirmed in animal studies. Studies reveal that camu camu is quite effective at blocking sugars (alpha-glucosidase) with only a few milligrams needed, and its blocking action against starch is much less effective (taking almost eight times as much camu camu required to block alpha-amylase). Camu camu contains a significant amount of quercetin, which is a well-known fat blocker (inhibiting pancreatic lipase). Brazilian researchers first confirmed the enzyme-inhibitor polyphenols in camu camu in 2010 and again in 2018 when they tested several tropical fruits for antioxidant and enzyme-inhibitor chemicals and actions.

In 2013, a Brazilian university research group published research about their investigation of the anti-obesity action of camu camu in a rat model of diet-induced obesity. After inducing obesity in rats, the rats were divided into two groups. One group was given camu camu fruit pulp daily for 12 weeks, and the control group received none. At the end of 12 weeks, researchers determined that the rats receiving camu camu reduced their weight by 31.7 percent, reduced their amount of body fat by 36.4 percent, and had lowered their glucose levels by 23 percent with increased insulin sensitivity. The researchers also reported a reduction in one of the main fat-produced pro-inflammatory chemicals, tumor necrosis factor alpha, by 12.7 percent. The elevation of this inflammatory chemical in obesity is one of the main reasons cancer risk increases with obesity. The group summarized their research saying: "Camu camu pulp was able to improve the biochemical profile of obesity in rats suggesting that this Amazonian fruit can be further used such a functional food ingredient in control of chronic diseases linked to obesity." These researchers surmised that their results were due to camu camu's high polyphenol content and remarked that the high amount of quercetin in the fresh fruit (400 mg/100 g fresh weight) was also responsible. Quercetin is a well-known and researched effective enzyme inhibitor and antioxidant.

Blood sugar levels rise for several hours after consuming a meal as sugars and carbs are absorbed during digestion. Brazilian researchers published a human study in 2017, which reported that when camu camu was taken with meals, it significantly decreased the rise of blood sugar after the meal in the healthy subjects they studied. The probable mechanism of action of the results documented was that the starches and sugars in the meal were not fully absorbed because of the fruit's enzyme-inhibiting actions that were noted in the 2013 study.

Other Brazilian researchers published a human study in 2015 that compared healthy subjects taking camu camu in capsules for 15 days and compared it to an equal number of subjects taking synthetic vitamin C, which they considered the control group. Their goal was to determine what benefits were derived from the vitamin C in comparison to camu camu in cholesterol, blood sugar, and vitamin C levels in the blood. Both capsules contained 320 milligrams of vitamin C. The researchers reported that there was a significant increase in serum levels of vitamin C (and much higher than the synthetic C group) and a significant drop in blood glucose and cholesterol values in the participants who received camu camu capsules. In the group that received synthetic vitamin C capsules, there was a significant decrease only in fasting glucose. This led researchers to summarize that camu camu capsules were more efficient at raising blood levels of vitamin C as well as lowering cholesterol and blood sugar levels than just synthetic vitamin C alone.

Newer research on camu camu's anti-obesity actions were published in 2018 by researchers in Canada. They described a different mechanism of action by which camu camu can help maintain a healthy weight. Some of the most cutting-edge research on the treatment and prevention of obesity is the result of a worldwide research initiative that has been conducted over the last 10 years, which is studying all of the many species of bacteria we have in our guts. All these bacteria reside in what is called the human gut microbiome. This large body of research reveals that many types of bacteria in our guts control a host of physiological functions in the body, including the promotion or reduction of inflammation, food metabolism and calorie absorption, insulin sensitivity, body-fat storage and fat burning, and a host of other functions. The gut microbiome is now considered a new organ that can be modified to treat and/or prevent obesity. Surprisingly, plant polyphenols have emerged in this research as the most effective and quickest way to modify the gut microbiome to encourage weight loss and make it easier to maintain a healthy weight. With the very high amounts of polyphenols in camu camu, it's not usual that researchers would choose this particular natural product to study how it could affect the gut microbiome.

These researchers studied camu camu in mice that were fed a high-sugar and high-fat diet to induce obesity. They reported that when mice were given camu camu with the obesity diet, it prevented weight gain, lowered fat accumulation, and reduced the metabolic inflammation that was documented in the control group (mice that didn't receive camu camu with the obesity diet). They also reported the mice receiving camu camu displayed improved glucose tolerance and insulin sensitivity and were also fully protected against hepatic steatosis (fatty liver), which developed in the control group due to the high-fat diet. In addition, they noted a remarkable change in bile acid production and composition in a manner that promoted calorie burning and weight loss.

They related these effects to the changes in the gut microbiome in the mice taking camu camu, rather than to the calorie-blocking enzyme inhibitors in camu camu. They noted that there was a significant reduction of bacterial species whose job it is to further extract calories, and an increase or bloom of other bacterial species that have been shown in microbiome research to encourage weight loss and reduce inflammation through several different mechanisms. One of the main mechanisms they noted was an increase of new chemicals (metabolites) produced by bacteria that increase fat and calorie burning as well as bile acid production, which have been well studied in the anti-obesity microbiome research to promote weight loss. To confirm these mechanisms, they took fecal samples (where all the bacterial resides) from the mice treated with camu camu as well as the nontreated obese mice and transplanted it into special germ/bacteria-free mice. They reported that mice colonized with fecal samples from camu camu–treated mice gained less weight and displayed higher fat and calorie burning than the mice colonized with fecal samples from the untreated mice, who all became obese like their transplant donors.

All of this microbiome research is rather technical and difficult to explain simply (and was the subject of an entire chapter on another rainforest plant book I recently finished). The remarkable news in all this new research is that we can either have a gut-bacteria profile that encourages weight gain or we can have a different ratio of bacteria that encourages weight loss and makes it easier to maintain a healthy weight. Polyphenols, and obviously the polyphenols in camu camu, have been shown to change the types and amounts of bacteria in our gut, which encourages weight loss. For more complete information on weight loss as it relates to the gut micro-biome, look for my book *Nature's Secret for Weight Loss*.

The research conducted on camu camu thus far indicates that this superfruit can positively affect obesity and diabetes through several mechanisms of actions. Research also indicates that camu camu could be used as an effective natural remedy both for treatment and preventative purposes. The substantial research discussed throughout this book reveals that if we maintain a healthy weight and healthy blood sugar levels, numerous diseases and conditions that are now known to be caused by obesity and diabetes can be prevented.

Cholesterol-Lowering Actions

As most are aware, the most important thing you can do to reduce your risk of developing heart disease is to keep your cholesterol at healthy levels. Many are unaware, however, that managing your free radicals is just as important. It is only when cholesterol becomes oxidized by free radicals that it increases the risk of clogged arteries (atherosclerosis). High oxidized cholesterol levels are more predictive of a possible heart attack than just measuring LDL cholesterol (the "bad" cholesterol). Having higher levels of oxidized cholesterol increase the risk of a heart attack by up to 400 percent.

Camu camu has demonstrated the ability through research to not only reduce the amount of oxidized cholesterol with its strong antioxidant abilities but also lower total cholesterol and triglycerides. The 2013 Brazilian animal study discussed earlier that documented camu camu's benefits for diabetes and weight loss also analyzed cholesterol levels in animals given camu camu with a high-fat and high-sugar diet. In addition to promoting weight gain, high-fat diets can also raise cholesterol levels. When rats were fed a high-fat and high-sugar diet along with camu camu, researchers reported that the rats reduced their cholesterol levels by 39.6 percent and triglycerides were also lowered by 40.6 percent. This was compared to the obese control group who had a 60 percent and 44 percent rise in cholesterol and triglycerides, respectively. HDL cholesterol (the "good" cholesterol) was increased in the rats fed camu camu by 12 percent. Researchers also noted an increase of fat eliminated in feces (by 50 percent) and in the liver (by 140 percent), which they attributed to the camu camu–fed rats being completely protected from fatty liver (hepatic steatosis).

In addition, the human study in 2015 that compared healthy subjects taking camu camu in capsules for 15 days discussed earlier also evaluated cholesterol levels in their research. The researchers reported that healthy subjects taking camu camu in capsules lowered total cholesterol by 21.8 percent and triglycerides by 5 percent. However, these study participants had normal cholesterol levels at the start of the study and didn't need lowering. The researchers noted that vitamin C has documented cholesterol-lowering actions through several mechanisms of action, as do other well-studied polyphenol compounds in camu camu and attributed their results to the combination of both.

Other Brazilian researchers published a study in 2014 that confirmed these same actions using a type 1 diabetes model in rats. Diabetic rats are often chosen simply because diabetes raises oxidative stress levels, which contribute to cholesterol increases. These researchers reported in the study that camu camu lowered cholesterol and triglycerides in amounts comparable to the previous study. They additionally confirmed that camu camu relieved oxidative stress and reduced the oxidation of fats and oxidized cholesterol in the animals. Three other animal studies concerning the cholesterol-lowering actions of camu camu have reported lowered cholesterol and triglycerides levels in their published research. See the reference section for a complete listing of the research discussed herein.

Again, reducing cholesterol, and especially oxidized cholesterol, is one of the best strategies, confirmed by years of research, to prevent the development of various heart diseases. It also helps explain why there has been a dramatic rise in the numbers of Americans developing heart disease with our much lower polyphenol diets. Managing your free radical levels by changing your diet to include a much higher amount of polyphenol-rich vegetables, fruits and whole grains will go a long way in reducing your risks of heat diseases. Changing lifestyle factors such as stopping smoking, maintaining a healthy weight, eliminating free-radical producing foods (fast foods and soda), and being more active also plays a role in protecting you from heart disease. And adding polyphenol-rich supplements like camu camu can help pick up the slack when we can't make all the healthy dietary and lifestyle changes we should to protect our hearts from disease.

Cancer Preventative Actions

It is well established that free radicals can damage DNA in various cells in our bodies which causes the DNA strand to break or rearranges the DNA coding. This DNA damage can result in a healthy cell mutating into a cancerous cell and ignoring the programed cell death code most cells are programmed for. For that reason, one of the main roles our natural built-in antioxidant system plays is to protect us from cancer by preventing the DNA damage free radicals can cause. This aspect is certainly a good reason to keep our antioxidant systems in good working order! Many plant polyphenol antioxidants, including those found in camu camu, have been reported to protect cells from mutating into cancerous cells, protect normal cellular signaling and coding, and some have even been documented with the ability to repair the DNA damage caused by free radicals. This has resulted in many studies around the world reporting that polyphenol-rich diets and as well as supplements rich in polyphenols provide cancer preventative actions. Camu camu, with its high natural antioxidant levels, is no exception.

Four animal and test-tube studies have confirmed camu camu's antimutagenic actions. In the *in vitro* studies, organ cells were pretreated with camu camu and introduced to various chemicals known to mutate them. Camu camu was shown to protect the cells from DNA strand breaks and mutation. A study published in 2014 reported these same *in vitro* results and also reported that the fruit juice evidenced an antiproliferative action (reduces or stops cancer cell growth) against liver cancer cells *in vitro*. They then tested the antimutagenic action in mice and reported that all dosages of camu camu they gave the animals provided beneficial antimutagenic actions. Other Brazilian researchers published a similar study with mice in 2019 and reported that camu camu was able to stop cells from mutating in various organs when the mice were introduced to several chemicals and drugs known to cause mutations through oxidative-stress processes. A university student in Peru wrote a thesis on their research on camu camu use in rats with colorectal cancer and reported that camu camu stopped the growth of tumors and reduced the inflammatory response.

Camu camu seems to be a popular study subject in Peruvian universities. Three doctoral theses on the antimutagenic abilities of camu camu fruit have been published by three different universities in Peru. Their research documented the fruit's ability to reduce cellular mutations in animals presented with various mutagenic drugs and substances by up to 90 percent. These researchers typically relate camu camu's antimutagenic actions to the fruit's vitamin C levels and antioxidant polyphenol profile. However, one researcher noted that the polyphenol, ellagic acid and the triterpenoid, betulinic acid, as well studied anticancer and antimutagenic compounds provided in significant amounts in camu camu.

There are no human studies indicating that the fruit is actually capable of treating cancer. Camu camu's main role for cancer is in prevention. Supporting our natural antioxidant system with camu camu, as described in this book, will provide benefits to protect healthy cells from turning into cancer cells. That antioxidants provide this benefit is well established by a significant body of research.

It is well established however, people who are battling cancer have a decreased antioxidant capacity, higher levels of damaging free radicals, and can be vitamin C deficient since their body's natural processes are trying to battle the cancer and are depleting these natural resources. These issues can be much worse while taking chemotherapy drugs, which usually increase oxidative stress to many organs to the point of toxicity. Taking camu camu as nutritional support while battling cancer can be a good strategy, and based on a growing understanding of polyphenol antioxidants, it may help reduce the negative side effects and toxicity to healthy cells and organs that chemotherapy drugs can cause.

Antimicrobial Actions

Since polyphenols effectively protect plants from various bacteria, fungus, mold, and viruses, it's not unusual that a high-polyphenol fruit like camu camu has been documented with the ability to kill or prevent the growth of these same disease-causing microbes. A dozen test-tube and animal studies confirm camu camu's ability to kill bacteria and candida. In addition to killing bacteria, two of these studies reported that a single compound in camu camu called 1-methyl malate was capable of reversing bacteria's drug resistance, which enabled standard antibiotic drugs to kill the bacteria in the test tube and animals.

Other studies confirm that camu camu juice is capable of killing several species of bacteria in the mouth linked to cavities, infections of the gums and teeth, and periodontal disease. These research groups reported camu camu was more effective than an antibiotic to kill mouth bacteria and surmised compounds in the juice were able to overcome the dental plaque and biofilm that mouth bacteria use to hide from antibiotics. Other research confirms than the anti-inflammatory nature of polyphenols, including the antibacterial polyphenols in camu camu that also reduce inflammation, are effective to reduce the swelling of chronically inflamed gums in periodontal disease.

Camu camu seems to be highly toxic to *Staphylococcus* and *Streptococcus* bacteria, at least *in vitro*, at very doses (as low as 0.08 mg/mL). Killing bacteria in the mouth is much like an *in vitro* test because the fruit or fruit juice comes in direct contact with the bacteria just like it does in the test tube. There haven't been any animal or human studies, however, reporting how drinking camu camu juice or taking camu camu powder in capsules will affect bacterial infections elsewhere inside the body and whether the antimicrobial compounds in camu camu can find the bacteria causing an infection inside the body and make an impact on it.

When camu camu was first launched into the American natural products market in the late 1990s, it was widely touted as a good antiviral for the flu virus as well as a host of other viruses. After reviewing all the published research on this fruit conducted over the last 30 years, I was surprised to see that not a single study has reported that camu camu was tested against any virus. Most of these initial antiviral claims were concerning camu camu's high vitamin C content as there were studies that indicated that high doses of vitamin C was helpful in speeding the recovery from the common flu virus. Over the last 20 years, research reports that vitamin C exerts a direct antiviral action that may provide specific protection against viral disease. The vitamin has been found to inactivate a wide spectrum of viruses as well as suppress viral replication and expression in infected cells. But interestingly, camu camu—the highest known source of vitamin C—has not been the subject of research to scientifically confirm if it might be capable of directly killing a virus in the same manner it kills bacteria.

Immune-Stimulant Actions

A Brazilian research group published a study in 2016 on the ability of camu camu to stimulate the immune system of fish (Nile tilapia). The fish were fed for five weeks using various dosages (0 to 500 milligrams of camu camu extract per kilogram of feed). Results after the five weeks revealed that fish receiving the camu camu at all dosages had significantly increased immunological responses by increasing white blood cells counts (lymphocytes, monocytes, neutrophils, and thrombocytes), as well as other measured immune-function increases.

Other university researchers in Brazil studied the immune-stimulation action of camu camu in rats in 2015. They fed rats camu camu for five days and then measured immune cells to compare them to the baseline numbers established before the intervention. Their results indicated that the number of mature lymphocytes (the body's main immune cell) in circulation increased by 100 percent and activity of phagocytes (natural killer cells, which remove foreign invaders like bacteria and viruses) was increased by 75.6 percent. The stimulation of phagocytic activity was noted in the reticuloendothelial system—a network of cells and tissues found throughout the body, especially in the blood, general connective tissue, spleen, liver, lungs, bone marrow, and lymph nodes.

Fertility-Enhancing Actions

Oxidative stress is a common culprit of several conditions associated with male fertility. High levels of reactive oxygen species (ROS) promote impairment of sperm quality mainly by decreasing motility and increasing the levels of DNA damage. Vitamin C deficiency has shown to cause male fertility issues in this regard as well, since it's a main player in our built-in antioxidant systems that is supposed to keep ROS at low levels. Within the testes are coiled masses of tubes called seminiferous tubules. These tubules are responsible for producing sperm cells through a process called spermatogenesis. Excess ROS can cause oxidative stress and mitochondrial dysfunction, resulting in low cellular energy in tubules, which interferes in spermatogenesis. Camu camu has been reported to aid in male fertility in two recent animal studies by relieving the oxidative stress and mitochondrial dysfunction and repair the sperm-creation process. Peruvian researchers studied camu camu in mice who were treated with low levels of radiation to create oxidative stress in the testes, which caused a significant reduction in sperm quality. Their 2019 research study reported that when they gave camu camu to the affected mice, the animals showed a significant recovery from the oxidative stress that altered the spermatogenesis process. This resulted in higher sperm levels.

Earlier, in 2013, researchers at a Peruvian university studied camu camu's effect on spermatogenesis in rats. They gave male rats camu camu for seven days and the rats were assessed for daily sperm production, stage of spermatogenic cycle, and antioxidant activity. They reported that camu camu increased the animals antioxidant levels and increased the ability of sperm cells to divide and multiply, which significantly increased the amount of sperm the animals produced daily.

CHAPTER 7

A Consumer Guide for Camu Camu

C amu camu supplements have been available for years and marketed as a vitamin C supplement. Hopefully, demand and use of camu camu will increase once consumers learn of this superfruit's many other benefits as outlined in this book. If consumers are looking for a natural remedy to heal their antioxidant systems and prevent the diseases associated with oxidative stress and the chronic inflammation it causes, camu camu has the highest antioxidant capacity over all other superfruits and should be a logical choice.

The Safety of Camu Camu

The long history of use of camu camu as a food has established that this natural tropical fruit is safe and well tolerated with few, if any, side effects. The animal and human research conducted on camu camu has not reported any signs of toxicity or negative side effects. A standard safety test was performed on camu camu in 2011 using both male and female mice. They evaluated the potential toxic effect of a range of different camu camu dosages and reported in both chronic (56 consecutive days) and acute (single high dosage in one day), and subacute (for 28 consecutive days) there was no evidence of toxicity or death. In the standard mutagenic test (to determine if camu camu could promote cell damage leading to cancer), researchers noted an antimutagenic and protective effect rather than a mutagenic effect. As reported in several studies, camu camu does prevent mutation of healthy cells into cancer cells.

Contraindications

❏ Large dosages (8 grams or more) of camu camu may cause loose stool and/or diarrhea.

Drug Interactions

❏ None reported.

Sources of Camu Camu

Most of the camu camu sold in the United States has been plantation grown, wild cultivated, or wild harvested in Brazil and Peru—the world's largest suppliers (and consumers) of camu camu products. Fresh camu camu fruit is too perishable to import into the United States. The camu camu products produced in South America include frozen or bottled fruit juice, dehydrated or freeze-dried juice, dehydrated or freeze-dried fruit pulp, and spray-dried fruit extracts. American suppliers and manufacturers typically import the available fruit powders to manufacture the camu camu supplements sold in retail and online health food stores.

Finding a Good Camu Camu Product

First, look for a certified organic source of camu camu. Countries in South America have different regulations about pesticides that may be allowed in food crops that may be banned in the United States.

Fruit Powders versus Juice Powders

There are three main types of camu camu powders that are sold in capsules, in tablets, or in bulk powder by the ounce and the pound. The first is a simple whole-fruit powder. The seeds are removed and the whole fruit is ground up and either freeze-dried or dehydrated, and the dried fruit is ground into a fine powder. This type of camu camu product is the best kind to purchase; it delivers comparable amounts of nutrients and beneficial compounds, with freeze-drying preserving a bit more than dehydration.

The second product is a pulp powder. The seeds and the fruit skin are removed and the pulp is either freeze-dried, dehydrated, or spray-dried. Since the fruit's skin contains a considerable amount of polyphenols that are responsible for the characteristic red color of the fruit, these types of powders contain much fewer polyphenols.

The next product (which I personally avoid) is a fruit juice powder. The fruit is juiced and the juice is then either freeze-dried or spray-dried. Approximately 40 percent of the fruit is left behind in the pressed skins, pulp, and seeds.

The real problem with fruit juice powder is that most of the polyphenols and a great deal of vitamin C have been left behind with the left-over pulp and skins after juicing. All "the stuff" left over after juicing a fruit is called "bagasse" in Brazil. Other countries typically call it agro-industrial waste since it has to be disposed of after the fruit is processed into juice. Brazilian and Peruvian juice manufacturers have discovered the polyphenol problem in their juices but instead of changing methods to get more polyphenols into their juice, they now just use the terminology of "by-product" instead of bagasse instead. See page 00 in the reference section under "Processing and Manufacturing Methods" to see the studies published on camu camu's bagasse or by-product. The fruit processing industry is industry is studying how they can either re-extract the bagasse utilizing a different method, or simply dry out the bagasse and grind it into a "flour" or powder to sell again as a polyphenol-rich camu camu "by-product." Reading this research certainly made me wonder just how many beneficial polyphenols actually remain in the juice when the fruit is processed into juice.

Recent research reports that the byproduct flour from camu camu showed a superior vitamin C and phenolic content than the juice powder (2.6 and 13.9 times, respectively). And, not surprisingly, the flour displayed greater antioxidant capacity than the pulp power (from 2.0 to 4.5 fold) when they tested it *in vitro* and in animals. The elevated polyphenol amounts in the flour are due to the camu camu seeds and skins being ground up with the other leftover stuff. Seeds and skin are an additional significant source of some of the same polyphenols found in the fruit and a few that aren't present in the fruit juice or pulp.

This camu camu flour may become an export product in the future and used in dietary supplements just as fruit, pulp, and fruit juice powders are sold now. This might be why so much research has been conducted on the byproduct flour. There has also been some recent quality research on the polyphenols and other active ingredients in camu camu seeds by researchers in Peru and Japan. Thus far, the seeds are reported with higher antimicrobial actions but slightly less antioxidant actions as the fruit. The seeds also contain compounds that are missing in the fruit that lower blood pressure levels. There is a distinct possibility that camu camu seed powder or seed oil products are on the horizon as well. A listing of the research conducted on camu camu seeds is shown in the reference section.

The least expensive camu camu products are spray-dried pulp and/or juice. Spray-drying is a standard method employed for many tropical fruits as well as medicinal plants. The fruit is chopped up, added to water and juiced (by mechanically squeezing or pressing). Then the juice is mixed typically 50% juice to 50% corn sugar (maltodextrin) and then another 5-15% of maltodextrin dextrose (more sugar) or guar gum is added in. This is then sprayed inside a hot rotating barrel that quickly evaporates off the water/moisture at very high temperature as it travels from the top of the barrel to the bottom, until only a powder remains. By volume, spray-dried extracts can be 75 percent or more corn sugar, but it is soluble in water and it is suitable to make capsule and tablet products with. Again, there is a significant loss of polyphenols in this process, since many polyphenols are water soluble, very delicate, and can't survive the high heat generated in this manufacturing method. Recent published studies on spray-dried camu camu pulp reported losses of polyphenols by 55, 72, and 87 percent compared to freeze-dried powders. See the reference section for a listing of these studies as well.

By far, the best product available (and more expensive) is a camu camu freeze-dried whole-fruit product. The second best is a whole-fruit dehydrated powder. These contain all of the vital nutrients and polyphenols contained in the plant, along with its beneficial fiber and pectin, with just the large amount of water (up to 90 percent) removed by freeze drying or dehydrating. This is the closest you can come to just eating the fresh fruit since fresh camu camu is not available here as a fresh fruit.

These products are available in bulk powders sold by the ounce or pound and can be found sold in capsules. The pulp powder products should be a light to medium tan color. The whole-fruit powders are a pink to a darker red or reddish-brown in color, which is coming from the dark-red fruit skins. These powders are intended to be stirred into water, juice, or smoothies and measured by the teaspoonful (1 teaspoon contains about 5 grams). They don't dissolve easily or completely in liquids, so a shaker cup or blender is recommended. The taste of these powders is quite tart with a strange aftertaste due to the high polyphenol content. Many say it is definitely an acquired taste, and others opt for capsules because they simply don't like the taste. Some just put the powder into another stronger-tasting juice or beverage to mask the camu camu taste.

If you are looking for a camu camu product in capsules or tablets, make sure to read the label closely and make sure it says "camu camu fruit" and doesn't use the words "juice" or "extract" in the Supplements Facts Box to obtain the highest polyphenol product. Also expect to see additives or flow agents as added ingredients on the label if the fruit was freeze-dried. The freeze-dried powder is difficult to encapsulate because it can reabsorb moisture from the air and becomes a bit sticky, and flow agents are required to get in into a capsule.

That brings us to the final issue with the problems of these manufactured spray-dried powders. A great deal of the vitamin C is lost in the high heat spray-dry process and even more is left behind in the by-product after juicing if it's a spray-dried juice extract. Some manufacturers are willing and capable of just adding cheap synthetic ascorbic acid to their extract products to replace the natural vitamin C that was lost by their processing. This has also been an issue with the so called "standardized extracts" of camu camu that are guaranteed to contain a specific amount of vitamin C. Some manufacturers of these products just add synthetic ascorbic acid to meet the promised amount of vitamin C rather than using more fruit to further concentrate camu camu to provide the natural version. In the U.S. tropical fruit import market, the most common adulterant affecting product quality of fruit powders is synthetic ascorbic acid and for that reason a special test was devised to identify this problem. When I see spray-dried standardized extracts that deliver more than 10 to 12 percent vitamin C (that doesn't cost at least eight to ten times more), it raises an eyebrow and makes me consider testing it for a synthetic C adulterant.

This brings us to the final point—if you want to find a good camu camu product, and/or if you choose an extract product, you need to choose a good, reputable U.S. manufacturer. Ethical manufacturers have a laboratory test they can use (if they choose to) that will determine if synthetic ascorbic acid is adulterating the camu camu powder they purchase to make their products.

With all these inherent issues with camu camu spray-dried powders, my personal choice is to stick with a natural freeze-dried or dehydrated camu camu whole fruit product and know that I'm getting all the natural compounds that were tested in this beneficial nutrient-dense tropical fruit without any human interference (and without all that added sugar). I also know that I have to pay more money for freeze-dried products, but at least I know what I am getting. My rule of thumb personally is to buy freeze-dried camu camu in bulk powders, but when I purchase camu camu capsules, I purchase dehydrated camu camu capsules because they're less expensive, they don't have all the fillers, and the polyphenol content is only slightly less than freeze-dried powders.

Where to Purchase Camu Camu

Camu camu products are sold under various brand names and are available in health food stores and through online retailers. Camu camu can also be found as an ingredient in various dietary supplements, including multi-vitamins. Camu camu's status as a "superfruit" has been well established in the market place and it is showing up in a growing number of functional foods and beverages in the natural products market. Quite a few companies offer good products, and the ones I've personally chosen for myself include Rainforest Pharmacy's dehydrated organic whole fruit camu camu in capsules and Feel Good Organic's organic freeze-dried whole camu camu powder in bulk. I'm not affiliated with or compensated by either company; I just buy their products for my own use after reviewing all the available products in the marketplace.

Suggested Dosages Camu Camu

Oftentimes, the dosages used and recommended for camu camu follow the dosages used for Vitamin C. The adult recommended dietary allowance (RDA) for vitamin C is 60-75 milligrams daily. However, most of the research reporting therapeutic benefits were using, on average, 500 to 1,000 milligrams daily in their studies. Therapeutic dosages of vitamin C for colds and flu, general illnesses, and debility are 1 to 5 grams daily. The average freeze-dried whole fruit camu camu powder contains around 600 to 750 milligrams of vitamin C per teaspoon of powder with dehydrated whole-fruit powders delivering around 550 to 600 milligrams per teaspoon.

For general prevention and to support your built-in antioxidant system, use 1 teaspoon of a freeze-dried or dehydrated camu camu powder daily in water, juice, a cup of hot tea, or blended into a smoothie. This amount is comparable to the dosages in the research on camu camu to address common free radical issues. You can substitute capsules for the powder if you prefer; just determine how many capsules are required to equal these recommended amounts (capsules sizes can vary).

If you want to try camu camu for weight loss, take 1 teaspoon of the freeze-dried or dehydrated powder 10 minutes before each meal with an 8-ounce glass of water. Camu camu works better for this purpose with the powder rather than capsules. If you want to substitute capsules anyway, avoid vegetable capsules and stick with gelatin capsules. Veggie cap products with camu camu won't deliver the enzyme-blocking polyphenols when the sugar and starch in meals are being digested in the stomach, since veggie caps don't dissolve well in stomach acid.

Therapeutic dosages in times of stress and illness, or if you have a diet or lifestyle that promotes more free radicals, use one teaspoon of the freeze-dried or dehydrated powder two or three times daily. You can substitute capsules for the powder if you prefer, just determine how many capsules are required to equal these recommended amounts (capsules sizes can vary).

If you have a cold, flu, sore throat or strep throat, dissolve a teaspoon of the powder in an 8-ounce cup of warm water, add the juice of half a lemon and 3 tablespoons of raw honey and sip slowly. Repeat several times daily. Adding one-half to a teaspoon of ground cinnamon to the cup will improve the flavor and cinnamon has a wealth of polyphenols and other natural compounds that are beneficial for reducing inflammation, fighting bacterial and viral infections, as well as free radicals.

Conclusion

We are currently in a healthcare crisis. Healthcare costs and health insurance rates have steadily risen as doctors' offices are jammed with patients, trying to treat diabetes, heart diseases, obesity, and a whole host of chronic diseases. The main goal of this book is to share new information that the underlying and contributing causes of these health problems are, in fact, largely caused by our failing antioxidants systems and how to naturally heal the natural processes in our antioxidant system to promote health and optimal wellness. The recent growth in the knowledge of free radicals and plant-based polyphenols is producing a medical revolution that promises a new age of health and disease management.

Tens of thousands of studies have been published in the last five years confirming that free radicals and the chronic inflammation and cellular damage they create are now a cause or contributing factor to many diseases and conditions, including type 2 diabetes and other metabolic diseases, clogged arteries and heart diseases, cancer, Alzheimer's disease and neurogenerative diseases, arthritis, autoimmune diseases, and even obesity. Oxidative stress and chronic inflammation from free radical damage are playing major roles in the development or progression of all these conditions. The link is even more clear in age-related chronic diseases and in aging itself.

The currently available drugs against chronic diseases are extremely expensive, minimally effective, and produce several side effects when taken for long period of time. My hope is that readers now have a clearer understanding of the problem and how natural and effective polyphenol and vitamin antioxidants, like those found in fruits and vegetables, as well as in camu camu, can be the natural solution to restore your antioxidant system to optimal levels to keep you protected from disease again.

References

This reference list was complete the day it was compiled; however, new studies are frequently published on this important medicinal plant. The citations below are listed in chronological order with the newest research listed first. Visit www.pubmed.gov to access the latest studies cataloged at the U.S. National Library of Medicine (PubMed). More information and periodic updated references on the research on camu camu can be found in the Rain-Tree Tropical Plant Database file for camu camu online at www.rain-tree.com/camu.htm.

Chapter 1. What is Camu Camu?

Akter, M., et al. "Nutritional compositions and health promoting phytochemicals of camu camu (*Myrciaria dubia*) fruit: a review." *Food Res. Int.* 2011; 44: 1728–1732.

Borges, L., et al., "Active compounds and medicinal properties of *Myrciaria* genus." *Food Chemistry.* 2014; 153: 224–233.

Bradfield R., et al. "Camu camu–a fruit high in ascorbic acid." *J. Am. Diet. Assoc.* 1964 Jan; 44: 28–30.

Castro, J., et al. "Variation of the contents of vitamin C and anthocyanins in *Myrciaria dubia* "camu camu." *Rev. Soc. Chem. Peru.* 2013; 79(4): 319–330.

Franco, M. R., et al. "Volatile composition of some Brazilian fruits: umbu-caja (*Spondias* citherea), camu camu (*Myrciaria dubia*), Araca-boi (*Eugenia stipitata*), and Cupuacu (*Theobroma grandiflorum*)." *J. Agric. Food Chem.* 2000; 48(4): 1263–5.

Grigio, M., et al. "Qualitative evaluation and biocompounds present in different parts of camu camu (*Myrciaria dubia*) fruit." *Afr. J. Food Sci.* 2017 May; 11: 124–129.

Quijano, C., et al. "Analysis of volatile compounds of camu camu (*Myrciaria dubia* (HBK) McVaugh) fruit isolated by different methods." *J. Essent. Oil. Res.* 2007; 19: 527–533.

Rodrigues, R., et al. "Antioxidant capacity of camu camu [*Myrciaria dubia* (H.B.K.) McVaugh] pulp." *Ernahrung. Nutr.* 2006; 30: 357–362.

Rodrigues, R., et al. "An Amazonian fruit with a high potential as a natural source of vitamin C: The camu camu (*Myrciaria dubia*)." *Fruits.* 2001; 56: 345–354.

Zanatta, C., et al. "Determination of anthocyanins from camu camu (*Myrciaria dubia*) by HPLC-PDA, HPLC-MS, and NMR." *J. Agric. Food Chem.* 2005 Nov 30; 53(24): 9531–5.

Zanatta, C., et al. "Carotenoid composition from the Brazilian tropical fruit camu–camu (*Myrciaria dubia*)." *Food Chem.* 2007; 4: 1526–1532.

Zapata, S., et al. "Camu camu *Myrciaria dubia* (HBK) McVaugh: Chemical composition of fruit." *J. Sci. Food Agricult.* 1993; 61(3): 349–351.

Chapter 2. Free Radicals and Antioxidants

Aruoma, O., et al. "Nutrition and health aspects of free radicals and antioxidants." *Food Chem. Toxicol.* 1994; 32: 671–83.

Bagchi, K., and Puri, S. "Free radicals and antioxidants in health and disease." *East Mediterranean Health J.* 1998; 4: 350–60.

Cheeseman, K., et al. "An introduction to free radical biochemistry." *Br. Med. Bull.* 1993 Jul; 49(3): 481–93.

Gupta, R., et al. "Oxidative stress and antioxidants in disease and cancer: A review." *Asian Pac. J. Cancer Prev.* 2014; 15: 4405–4409.

Halliwell, B., and Gutteridge, J. "*Free radicals in biology and medicine.*" 4th ed. Oxford, UK: Clarendon Press; 2007.

He, L., et al. "Antioxidants maintain cellular redox homeostasis by elimination of reactive oxygen species." *Cell. Physiol. Biochem.* 2017; 44: 532–553.

Housset, B. "Biochemical aspects of free radicals metabolism." *Bull. Eur. Physiopathol. Respir.* 1987 Jul–Aug; 23(4): 287–90.

Lobo, V., et al. "Free radicals, antioxidants and functional foods: Impact on human health." *Pharmacogn. Rev.* 2010 Jul–Dec; 4(8): 118–126.

Matsuda, M., et al. "Increased oxidative stress in obesity: implications for metabolic syndrome, diabetes, hypertension, dyslipidemia, atherosclerosis, and cancer." *Obes. Res. Clin. Pract.* 2013; 7: e330–e341.

References

Pham-Huv, L., et al. "Free radicals, antioxidants in disease and health." *Int. J. Biomed. Sci.* 2008 Jun; 4(2): 89–96.

Rock, C., "Update on biological characteristics of the antioxidant micronutrients - Vitamin C, Vitamin E and the carotenoids." *J. Am. Diet. Assoc.* 1996; 96: 693–702.

Sagnoun, Z., et al. "Free radicals and antioxidants: human physiology, pathology and therapeutic aspects." *Therapie.* 1997 Jul–Aug; 52(4): 251–70.

Valko, M., et al. "Free radicals and antioxidants in normal physiological functions and human disease." *Review. Int. J. Biochem. Cell. Biol.* 2007; 39: 44–84.

Xu, D., et al. "Natural antioxidants in foods and medicinal plants: extraction, assessment and resources." *Int. J. Mol. Sci.* 2017 Jan; 18(1): 96.

Young, I., and Woodside, J. "Antioxidants in health and disease." *J. Clin. Pathol.* 2001; 54: 176–186.

Chapter 3. The Benefits of Vitamin C

Ali, S., et al. "Understanding oxidants and antioxidants: Classical team with new players." *J. Food Biochem.* 2020 Jan; 13145. (ahead of print)

Amr, M., et al. "Efficacy of vitamin C as an adjunct to fluoxetine therapy in pediatric major depressive disorder: A randomized, double-blind, placebo-controlled pilot study." *Nutr. J.* 2013; 12: 31.

Ashor, A., et al. "Effect of vitamin C on endothelial function in health and disease: a systematic review and meta-analysis of randomised controlled trials." *Atherosclerosis.* 2014 Jul; 235(1): 9–20.

Baxter, R., et al. "Vitamin C and glaucoma." *J. Am. Optom. Assoc.* 1988 Jun; 59(6): 438.

Carr, A., and Maggini, S. "Vitamin C and immune function." *Nutrients.* 2017 Nov; 9(11): E1211.

Carr, A., "Synthetic or food-derived vitamin C–are they equally bioavailable?" *Nutrients.* 2013 Nov; 5(11): 4284–4304.

Chen, K., et al. "Vitamin C suppresses oxidative lipid damage *in vivo*, even in the presence of iron overload." *Am. J. Physiol. Endocrinol. Metab.* 2000; 279: E1406–12.

Choi, H., et al. "Vitamin C intake and the risk of gout in men: a prospective study." *Arch. Intern. Med.* 2009 Mar; 169(5): 502–7.

Colagar, A., et al. "Ascorbic acid in human seminal plasma: determination and its relationship to sperm quality." *J. Clin. Biochem. Nutr.* 2009 Sep; 45(2): 144–9.

Cosgrove, M., et al. "Dietary nutrient intakes and skin-aging appearance among middle-aged American women." *Am. J. Clin. Nutr.* 2007; 86: 1225–1231.

de Oliveira, I., et al. "Effects of oral vitamin C supplementation on anxiety in students: a double-blind, randomized, placebo-controlled trial." *Pak. J. Biol. Sci.* 2015 Jan; 18(1): 11–8.

Fidanza, A., et al. "Therapeutic action of vitamin C on cholesterol metabolism." *Boll. Soc. Ital. Biol. Sper.* 1979 Mar; 55(6): 553–8.

Fiorani, M., et al. "Mitochondrial reactive oxygen species: The effects of mitochondrial ascorbic acid vs untargeted and mitochondria-targeted antioxidants." *Int. J. Radiat. Biol.* 2020 Jan 24: 1–25.

Gale, C., et al. "Cognitive impairment and mortality in a cohort of elderly people." *BMJ.* 1996 Mar; 312(7031): 608–11.

Gautam, M., et al. "Role of antioxidants in generalised anxiety disorder and depression." *Indian J. Psychiatry.* 2012; 54: 244–247.

Goodwin, J., et al. "Association between nutritional status and cognitive functioning in a healthy elderly population." *JAMA.* 1983 Jun; 249(21): 2917–21.

Hagel, A., et al. "Intravenous infusion of ascorbic acid decreases serum histamine concentrations in patients with allergic and non-allergic diseases." *Naunyn. Schmiedebergs Arch. Pharmacol.* 2013 Sep; 386(9): 789–93.

Hemila, H. "Vitamin C and common cold-induced asthma: a systematic review and statistical analysis." *Allergy Asthma Clin. Immunol.* 2013 Nov; 9(1): 46.

Hemila, H., et al. "Vitamin C for preventing and treating the common cold." *Cochrane Database Syst Rev.* 2013 Jan 31; (1): CD000980.

Huijskens, M., et al. "Technical advance: ascorbic acid induces development of double-positive T cells from human hematopoietic stem cells in the absence of stromal cells." *J. Leukoc. Biol.* 2014 Dec; 96(6): 1165–75.

Hysi, P., et al. "Ascorbic acid metabolites are involved in intraocular pressure control in the general population." *Redox Biol.* 2019 Jan; 20: 349–353.

Johnston, C., et al. "Antihistamine effect of supplemental ascorbic acid and neutrophil chemotaxis." *J. Am. Coll. Nutr.* 1992 Apr; 11(2): 172–6.

Juraschek, S., et al. "Effect of oral vitamin C supplementation on serum uric acid: a meta-analysis of randomized controlled trials." *Arthritis Care Res.* 2011 Sep; 63(9): 1295–306.

Juraschek, S., et al. "Effects of vitamin C supplementation on blood pressure: a meta-analysis of randomized controlled trials." *Am. J. Clin. Nutr.* 2012 May; 95(5): 1079–88.

Kim, S., et al. "Consumption of high-dose vitamin C (1250 mg per day) enhances functional and structural properties of serum lipoprotein to improve anti-oxidant, anti-atherosclerotic, and anti-aging effects via regulation of anti-inflammatory microRNA." *Food Funct.* 2015 Nov; 6(11): 3604–12.

Knekt, P., et al. "Antioxidant vitamins and coronary heart disease risk: a pooled analysis of 9 cohorts." *Am. J. Clin. Nutr.* 2004 Dec; 80(6): 1508–20.

Kocot, J., et al. "Does vitamin C influence neurodegenerative diseases and psychiatric disorders?" *Nutrients.* 2017 Jun; 9(7): E659.

Kurti, S., et al. "Improved lung function following dietary antioxidant supplementation in exercise-induced asthmatics." *Respir. Physiol. Neurobiol.* 2016 Jan; 220: 95–101.

Luck, M., et al. "Ascorbic acid and fertility." *Biol. Reprod.* 1995 Feb; 52(2): 262–6.

Mao, X., and Yao, G. "Effect of vitamin C supplementations on iron deficiency anemia in Chinese children." *Biomed. Environ. Sci.* 1992 Jun; 5(2): 125–9.

McArdle, F., et al. "UVR-induced oxidative stress in human skin *in vivo*: effects of oral vitamin C supplementation." *Free Radic. Biol. Med.* 2002; 33: 1355–1362.

McRae, M. "Vitamin C supplementation lowers serum low-density lipoprotein cholesterol and triglycerides: a meta-analysis of 13 randomized controlled trials." *J. Chiropr. Med.* 2008 Jun; 7(2): 48–58.

Mikirova, N., et al. "The effect of high dose IV vitamin C on plasma antioxidant capacity and level of oxidative stress in cancer patients and healthy subjects." *J. Orthomol. Med.* 2007; 22: 3.

Moser, M., et al. "Vitamin C and heart health: A review based on findings from epidemiologic studies." *Int. J. Mol. Sci.* 2016 Aug 12; 17(8).

Nauman, G., et al. "Systematic review of intravenous ascorbate in cancer clinical trials." *Antioxidants.* 2018 Jul; 7(7): E89.

Ngo, B., et al. "Targeting cancer vulnerabilities with high-dose vitamin C." 2019 Apr; 19: 271–282.

Padayatty, S., et al. "Vitamin C as an antioxidant: Evaluation of its role in disease prevention." *J. Am. Coll. Nutr.* 2003; 22: 18–35.

Paleologos, M., et al. "Cohort study of vitamin C intake and cognitive impairment." *Am. J. Epidemiol.* 1998 Jul; 148(1): 45–50.

Popovic, L., et al. "Influence of vitamin C supplementation on oxidative stress and neutrophil inflammatory response in acute and regular exercise." *Oxid. Med. Cell. Longev.* 2015 Feb; 2015: 295497.

Rafiee, B., et al. "Comparing the effectiveness of dietary vitamin C and exercise interventions on fertility parameters in normal obese men." *Urol. J.* 2016 Apr; 13(2): 2635–9.

Ramdas, W., et al. "The effect of vitamins on glaucoma: A systematic review and meta-analysis." *Nutrients.* 2018 Mar; 10(3): E359.

Ran, L., et al. "Extra dose of vitamin C based on a daily supplementation shortens the common cold: a meta-analysis of 9 randomized controlled trials." *Biomed. Res. Int.* 2018 Jul; 2018: 1837634.

Retsky, K., et al. "Ascorbic acid oxidation product(s) protect human low density lipoprotein against atherogenic modification. Anti-rather than prooxidant activity of vitamin C in the presence of transition metal ions." *J. Biol. Chem.* 1993; 268: 1304–9.

Rubio-Lopez, N., et al. "Nutrient intake and depression symptoms in Spanish children: The ANIVA Study." *Int. J. Environ. Res. Public Health.* 2016; 13: 352.

Sanchez-Quesada, J., et al. "Ascorbic acid inhibits the increase in low-density lipoprotein (LDL) susceptibility to oxidation and the proportion of electronegative LDL induced by intense aerobic exercise." *Coron. Artery Dis.* 1998; 9(5): 249–55.

Schencking, M., et al. "Intravenous vitamin C in the treatment of shingles: results of a multicenter prospective cohort study." *Med. Sci. Monit.* 2012 Apr; 18(4): CR215–24.

Taddei, S., et al. "Vitamin C improves endothelium-dependent vasodilation by restoring nitric oxide activity in essential hypertension." *Circulation* 1998; 97: 2222–9.

Tang, L. "Comparative study of the bioavailability of ascorbic acid in commercially produced products." Dissertation 1995. University of Pennsylvania, Department of Chemistry.

Turley, S., et al. "The role of ascorbic acid in the regulation of cholesterol metabolism and in the pathogenesis of atherosclerosis." *Atherosclerosis.* 1976 Jul–Aug; 24(1-2): 1–18.

Volbracht, C., et al. "Intravenous vitamin C in the treatment of allergies: an interim subgroup analysis of a long-term observational study." *J. Int. Med. Res.* 2018 Sep; 46(9): 3640–3655.

Wang, K., et al. "Role of vitamin C in skin diseases." *Front. Physiol.* 2018 Jul; 9: 819.

Ye, Z., et al. "Antioxidant vitamins intake and the risk of coronary heart disease: meta-analysis of cohort studies." *Eur. J. Cardiovasc. Prev. Rehabil.* 2008 Feb; 15(1): 26–34.

Zhang, M., et al. "Vitamin C provision improves mood in acutely hospitalized patients." *Nutrition.* 2011; 27: 530–533.

References

Chapter 4. The Power of Polyphenols

An, J., et al. "Natural products for treatment of osteoporosis: The effects and mechanisms on promoting osteoblast-mediated bone formation." *Life Sci.* 2016 Feb; 147: 46–58.

Anhe, F., et al. "Polyphenols and type 2 diabetes: A prospective review." *Pharma. Nutrition.* 2013; 1: 105–114.

Ashok, B., et al. "The aging paradox: Free radical theory of aging." *Exp. Gerontol.* 1999; 34: 293–303.

Assini, E., et al. "Antiobesity effects of anthocyanins in preclinical and clinical studies." *Oxid. Med. Cell. Longev.* 2017; 2017: 2740364.

Bijak, M., et al. "Popular naturally occurring antioxidants as potential anticoagulant drugs." *Chem. Biol. Interact.* 2016 Sep; 257: 35–45.

Bijak, M., et al. "Polyphenol compounds belonging to flavonoids inhibit activity of coagulation factor X." *Int. J. Biol. Macromol.* 2014 Apr; 65: 129–35.

Callejo, M., et al. "Impact of nutrition on pulmonary arterial hypertension." *Nutrients.* 2020 Jan; 12(1): E169.

Carrasco-Pozo, C., et al. "Quercetin and epigallocatechin gallate in the prevention and treatment of obesity: from molecular to clinical studies." *J. Med. Food.* 2019 Aug; 22(8): 753–770.

Correa, T., et al. "The two-way polyphenols-microbiota interactions and their effects on obesity and related metabolic diseases." *Front. Nutr.* 2019 Dec; 6: 188.

Chen, Y., et al. "Polyphenols and oxidative stress in atherosclerosis-related ischemic heart disease and stroke." *Oxid. Med. Cell. Longev.* 2017; 2017: 8526438.

Davinelli, S., et al. "Cytoprotective polyphenols against chronological skin aging and cutaneous photodamage." *Curr. Pharm. Des.* 2018; 24(2): 99–105.

Dilberger, B., et al. "Polyphenols and metabolites enhance survival in rodents and nematodes-impact of mitochondria." *Nutrients.* 2019 Aug; 11(8): E1886.

Dryden, G., et al. "Polyphenols and gastrointestinal diseases." *Curr. Opin. Gastroenterol.* 2006 Mar; 22(2): 165–170.

Grosso, G., et al. "Dietary polyphenol intake and risk of type 2 diabetes in the Polish arm of the health, alcohol and psychosocial factors in eastern Europe (HAPIEE) study." *Br. J. Nutr.* 2017 Jul; 118(1): 60–68.

Gupta, R., et al. "Oxidative stress and antioxidants in disease and cancer: a review." *Asian Pac. J. Cancer Prev.* 2014; 15: 4405–4409.

Hua, J., et al. "Dietary polyphenols turn fat "brown": A narrative review of the possible mechanisms." *Trends Food Sci. Technol.* 2020 Mar; 97: 221–232.

Hussain, T., et al. "Oxidative stress and inflammation: what polyphenols can do for us? *Oxid. Med. Cell. Longev.* 2016; 2016: 7432797.

Karim, N., et al. "An increasing role of polyphenols as novel therapeutics for Alzheimer's: A review." *Med. Chem.* 2019; Nov 5. (ahead of print)

Kim, Y., et al. "Polyphenols and glycemic control." *Nutrients.* 2016 Jan; 8(1): 17.

Li, A., et al. "Resources and biological activities of natural polyphenols." *Nutrients.* 2014 Dec; 6(12): 6020–6047.

Liu, J., et al. "Beneficial effects of dietary polyphenols on high-fat diet-induced obesity linking with modulation of gut microbiota." *J. Agric. Food Chem.* 2020 Jan; 68(1): 33–47.

Majidinia, M., et al. "Targeting miRNAs by polyphenols: Novel therapeutic strategy for aging." *Biochem. Pharmacol.* 2019 Nov 1: 113688. (ahead of print)

Marchesi, J., et al. "The gut microbiota and host health: a new clinical frontier." *Gut.* 2016 Feb; 65(2): 330–9.

Marin, L., et al. "Bioavailability of dietary polyphenols and gut microbiota metabolism: antimicrobial properties." *Biomed. Res. Int.* 2015; 2015: 905215.

Mir, S., et al. "Understanding the role of active components from plant sources in obesity management." *J. Saudi. Soc. Agric. Sci.* 2019; 18: 168–176.

Niedzwiecki, A., et al. "Anticancer efficacy of polyphenols and their combinations." *Nutrients.* 2016 Sep; 8(9): 552.

Pacheco-Ordaz, R., et al. "Effect of phenolic compounds on the growth of selected probiotic and pathogenic bacteria." *Lett. Appl. Microbiol.* 2018 Jan; 66(1): 25–31.

Poti, F., et al. "Polyphenol health effects on cardiovascular and neurodegenerative disorders: a review and meta-analysis." *Int. J. Mol. Sci.* 2019 Jan; 20(2): 351.

Ribeiro da Silva, L., et al. "Quantification of bioactive compounds in pulps and by-products of tropical fruits from Brazil." *Food Chem.* 2014 Jan; 143: 398–404.

Rienks, J., et al. "Association of polyphenol biomarkers with cardiovascular disease and mortality risk: A systematic review and meta-analysis of observational studies." *Nutrients.* 2017 Apr; 9(4): 415.

Rowland, I., et al. "Gut microbiota functions: metabolism of nutrients and other food components." *Eur. J. Nutr.* 2018 Feb; 57(1): 1–24.

Russo, G., et al. "Mechanisms of aging and potential role of selected polyphenols in extending healthspan." *Biochem. Pharmacol.* 2019 Nov 21: 113719.

Shahidi, F., et al. "Phenolics and polyphenolics in foods, beverages and spices: Antioxidant activity and health effects – A review." *J. Funct. Foods* 2015; 18: 820–897.

References

Silva, R., et al. "Polyphenols from food and natural products: neuroprotection and safety." *Antioxidants.* 2020 Jan; 9(1): E61.

Silvester, A., et al. "Dietary polyphenols and their roles in fat browning." *J. Nutr. Biochem.* 2019 Feb; 64: 1–12.

Tangney, C., et al. "Polyphenols, inflammation, and cardiovascular disease." *Curr. Atheroscler. Rep.* 2013 May; 15(5): 324.

Williamson, G., et al. "The role of polyphenols in modern nutrition." *Nutr. Bull.* 2017 Sep; 42(3): 226–235.

Xiao, J., et al. "Dietary polyphenols and type 2 diabetes: current insights and future perspectives." *Curr. Med. Chem.* 2015; 22(1): 23–38.

Zang, H., et al. "Dietary polyphenols, oxidative stress and antioxidant and anti-inflammatory effects." *Curr. Opin. Food Sci.* 216 Apr; 8: 33–42.

Zhou, Y., et al. "Natural polyphenols for prevention and treatment of cancer." *Nutrients.* 2016 Aug; 8(8): 515.

Chapter 5. How Camu Camu Prevents Disease

Bungau, S., et al. "Health benefits of polyphenols and carotenoids in age-related eye diseases." *Oxid. Med. Cell. Longev.* 2019; 2019: 9783429.

Cao, H., et al. "Dietary polyphenols and type 2 diabetes: human study and clinical trial." *Crit. Rev. Food Sci. Nutr.* 2019; 59(20): 3371–3379.

Ceriello, A., et al. "Possible role of oxidative stress in the pathogenesis of hypertension." *Diabetes Care.* 2008 Feb; 31 Suppl 2: S181–4.

Cheng, Y., et al. "Polyphenols and oxidative stress in atherosclerosis-related ischemic heart disease and stroke." *Oxid. Med. Cell. Longev.* 2017; 2017: 8526438.

De Bruyne, T., et al. "Dietary polyphenols targeting arterial stiffness: interplay of contributing mechanisms and gut microbiome-related metabolism." *Nutrients.* 2019 Mar; 11(3): 578.

Dunmore, S., et al. "The role of adipokines in -cell failure of type 2 diabetes." *J. Endocrinol.* 2013 Jan; 216(1): T37–45.

Ellulu, M., et al. "Obesity and inflammation: the linking mechanism and the complications." *Arch. Med. Sci.* 2017; 13(4): 851–863.

Engin, A., et al. "The pathogenesis of obesity-associated adipose tissue inflammation." *Adv. Exp. Med. Biol.* 2017; 960: 221–245.

Fernandez-Sanchez, A., et al. "Inflammation, oxidative stress, and obesity." *Int. J. Mol. Sci.* 2011; 12(5): 3117–3132.

Figueira, I., et al. "Polyphenols beyond barriers: a glimpse into the brain." *Curr. Neuropharmacol.* 2017 May; 15(4): 562–594.

Grootaert, C., et al. "Cell systems to investigate the impact of polyphenols on cardiovascular health." *Nutrients.* 2015 Nov; 7(11): 9229–9255.

Gupta, R., et al. "Oxidative stress and antioxidants in disease and cancer: a review." *Asian Pac. J. Cancer Prev.* 2014; 15: 4405–4409.

Hussain, T., et al. "Oxidative stress and inflammation: what polyphenols can do for us?" *Oxid. Med. Cell. Longev.* 2016; 2016: 7432797.

Ighodaro, O., et al. "Molecular pathways associated with oxidative stress in diabetes mellitus." *Biomed. Pharmacother.* 2018; 108: 656–662.

Jan, F., et al. "Mitochondria-centric review of polyphenol bioactivity in cancer models." *Antioxid. Redox. Signal.* 2018 Dec; 29(16): 1589–1611.

Jayasena, T., et al. "The role of polyphenols in the modulation of sirtuins and other pathways involved in Alzheimer's disease." *Age. Res. Rev.* 2013; 12: 867–883.

Kim, Y., et al. "Polyphenols and glycemic control." *Nutrients.* 2016 Jan; 8(1): 17.

Koch, W. "Dietary polyphenols—important non-nutrients in the prevention of chronic noncommunicable diseases. a systematic review." *Nutrients.* 2019 May; 11(5): 1039.

Kwon, O., et al. "Inhibition of the intestinal glucose transporter GLUT2 by flavonoids." *FASEB J.* 2007; 21: 366–377.

Li, S., et al. "The potential and action mechanism of polyphenols in the treatment of liver diseases." *Oxid. Med. Cell. Longev.* 2018; 2018: 8394818.

Liang, W., et al. "The potential of adipokines as biomarkers and therapeutic agents for vascular complications in type 2 Diabetes mellitus." *Cytokine Grow. Fact. Rev.* 2019 Aug; 48: 32–39.

Matsuda M, et al. "Increased oxidative stress in obesity: implications for metabolic syndrome, diabetes, hypertension, dyslipidemia, atherosclerosis, and cancer." *Obes. Res. Clin. Pract.* 2013; 7: e330–e341.

Mattera, R., et al. "Effects of polyphenols on oxidative stress-mediated injury in cardiomyocytes." *Nutrients.* 2017 May; 9(5): 523.

Mihaylova, D., et al. "Polyphenols as suitable control for obesity and diabetes." *Open Biotech. J.* 2010 Sept; 12: 219–228.

Naoi, M., et al. "Mitochondria in neuroprotection by phytochemicals: bioactive polyphenols modulate mitochondrial apoptosis system, function and structure." *Int. J. Mol. Sci.* 2019 May; 20(10): 2451.

Pan, M., et al., "Anti-inflammatory activity of natural dietary flavonoids." *Food Funct.* 2010; 1; 15-31.

Pasinetti, G., et al. "The role of the gut microbiota in the metabolism of polyphenols as characterized by gnotobiotic mice." *J. Alzheimer. Dis.* 2018; 63(2): 409–421.

Radak, Z., et al., "Age-associated neurodegeneration and oxidative damage to lipids, proteins and DNA." *Mol. Asp. Med.* 2011; 32: 305-315.

Rienks, J., et al. "Polyphenol exposure and risk of type 2 diabetes: dose-response meta-analyses and systematic review of prospective cohort studies." *Am. J. Clin. Nutr.* 2018; 108: 49–61.

Silveira, A., et al. "The action of polyphenols in Diabetes mellitus and Alzheimer's disease: a common agent for overlapping pathologies." *Curr. Neuropharmacol.* 2019 Jul; 17(7): 590–613.

Serino, A., and Salazar, G. "Protective role of polyphenols against vascular inflammation, aging and cardiovascular disease." *Nutrients.* 2018 Dec; 11(1): E53.

Tressera-Rimbau, A., et al. "Dietary polyphenols in the prevention of stroke." *Oxid. Med. Cell. Longev.* 2017; 2017: 7467962.

Vauzour, D., et al. "Polyphenols and human health: prevention of disease and mechanisms of action." *Nutrients.* 2010 Nov; 2(11): 1106–1131.

Wang, X., et al. "Flavonoid intake and risk of CVD: a systematic review and meta-analysis of prospective cohort studies." *Br. J. Nutr.* 2014 Jan; 111(1): 1–11.

Woo, C., et al. "Mitochondrial dysfunction in adipocytes as a primary cause of adipose tissue inflammation." *Diabetes Metab. J.* 2019 Jun; 43(3): 247256.

Yahfoufi, N., et al. "The immunomodulatory and anti-inflammatory role of polyphenols." *Nutrients.* 2018 Nov; 10(11): 1618.

Chapter 6. The Research on Camu Camu

Anti-Aging and AGE-Inhibitor Actions

Azevedo, J., et al. "Neuroprotective effects of dried camu camu (*Myrciaria dubia* HBK McVaugh) residue in *C. elegans.*" *Food Res. Intl.* 2015 Jul; 73: 135–141.

Fujita, A., et al. "Evaluation of phenolic-linked bioactives of camu camu (*Myrciaria dubia* Mc. Vaugh) for antihyperglycemia, antihypertension, antimicrobial properties and cellular rejuvenation." *Food Res. Int.* 2015; 77(Part 2): 194–203.

Muthenna, P., et al. "Ellagic acid, a new antiglycating agent: its inhibition of Nε-(carboxymethyl)lysine." *Biochem. J.* 2012 Feb; 442(1): 221–30.

Raghu, G., et al. "Attenuation of diabetic retinopathy in rats by ellagic acid through inhibition of AGE formation." *J. Food Sci. Technol.* 2017 Jul; 54(8): 2411–2421.

Rahimi, V., et al. "Ellagic acid dose and time-dependently abrogates d-galactose-induced animal model of aging: Investigating the role of PPAR-γ." *Life Sci.* 2019 Sep; 232: 116595.

Rahimi, V., et al. "Ellagic acid reveals promising anti-aging effects against d-galactose-induced aging on human neuroblastoma cell line, SH-SY5Y: A mechanistic study." *Biomed. Pharmacother.* 2018 Dec; 108: 1712–1724.

Rios, J., et al. "A pharmacological update of ellagic acid." *Planta Med.* 2018 Oct; 84(15): 1068–1093.

Suantawee, T., et al. "Protective effect of cyanidin against glucose- and methylglyoxal-induced protein glycation and oxidative DNA damage." *Int. J. Biol. Macromol.* 2016 Dec; 93(Pt A): 814–821.

Thilavech, T., et al. "Cyanidin-3-rutinoside attenuates methylglyoxal-induced protein glycation and DNA damage via carbonyl trapping ability and scavenging reactive oxygen species." *BMC Complement. Altern. Med.* 2016 May 23; 16: 138.

Anti-Inflammatory Actions

Allam, G., et al. "Ellagic acid alleviates adjuvant induced arthritis by modulation of pro- and anti-inflammatory cytokines." *Cent. Eur. J. Immunol.* 2016; 41(4): 339–349.

Chen, P., et al. "Antioxidative, anti-inflammatory and anti-apoptotic effects of ellagic acid in liver and brain of rats treated by D-galactose." *Sci. Rep.* 2018 Jan 23; 8(1): 1465.

Derosa, G., et al. "Ellagic acid and its role in chronic diseases." *Adv. Exp. Med. Biol.* 2016; 928: 473–479.

Fikry, E., et al. "Caffeic acid and ellagic acid ameliorate adjuvant-induced arthritis in rats via targeting inflammatory signals, chitinase-3-like protein-1 and angiogenesis." *Biomed. Pharmacother.* 2019 Feb; 110: 878–886.

Gupta, S., et al. "Inflammation, a double-edge sword for cancer and other age-related diseases." *Front. Immunol.* 2018 Sep; 9: 2160.

Huimin, D., et al. "Protective effect of betulinic acid on Freund's complete adjuvant-induced arthritis in rats." *J. Biochem. Mol. Toxicol.* 2019 Sep; 33(9): e22373.

Inoue, T., et al. "Tropical fruit camu camu (*Myrciaria dubia*) has anti-oxidative and anti-inflammatory properties." *J. Cardiol.* 2008 Oct; 52(2): 127–32.

Langley, P., et al. "Antioxidant and associated capacities of camu camu (*Myrciaria dubia*): a systematic review." *J. Altern. Complement. Med.* 2015 Jan; 21(1): 8–14.

Lin, Z., et al. "The protective effect of ellagic acid (EA) in osteoarthritis: An *in vitro* and *in vivo* study." *Biomed. Pharmacother.* 2020 Feb; 125: 109845.

References

Murphy, M., et al. "The polyphenol ellagic acid exerts anti-inflammatory actions via disruption of store-operated calcium entry (SOCE) pathway activators and coupling mediators." *Eur. J. Pharmacol.* 2020 Feb 23: 173036.

Ou, Z., et al. "Anti-inflammatory effect and potential mechanism of betulinic acid on λ-carrageenan-induced paw edema in mice." *Biomed. Pharmacother.* 2019 Oct; 118: 109347.

Rios, J., and Manez, S. "New pharmacological opportunities for betulinic acid." *Planta Med.* 2018 Jan; 84(1): 8–19.

Rios, J., et al. "A pharmacological update of ellagic acid." *Planta Med.* 2018 Oct; 84(15): 1068–1093.

Serrano, A., et al. "Bioactive compounds and extracts from traditional herbs and their potential anti-inflammatory health effects." *Medicines.* 2018 Jul; 5(3): E76.

Wang, X., et al. "Protective effects of betulinic acid on intestinal mucosal injury induced by cyclophosphamide in mice." *Pharmacol. Rep.* 2019 Oct; 71(5): 929–939.

Yazawa, K., et al. "Anti-inflammatory effects of seeds of the tropical fruit camu camu (*Myrciaria dubia*)." *J. Nutr. Sci. Vitaminol.* 2011; 57(1): 104–7.

Antimicrobial Actions

Alimirzaee, P., et al. "L-methyl malate from *Berberis integerrima* fruits enhances the antibacterial activity of ampicillin against *Staphylococcus aureus.*" *Phytother Res.* 2009 Jun; 23(6): 797–800.

Camere-Colarossi, R., et al. "Antibacterial activity of *Myrciaria dubia* (camu camu) against *Streptococcus mutans* and *Streptococcus sanguinis.*" *Asian Pacif. J. Tropical Biomed.* 2016; 6(9): 740–744.

Castillo-Carranza, C., "*In vitro* inhibitory effect of *Myrciaria dubia* "camu camu" on *Staphylococcus aureus* and *Candida albicans.*" Thesis 2013. National University of Trujillo. Trujillo, Peru.

Fujita, A., et al. "Evaluation of phenolic-linked bioactives of camu camu (*Myrciaria dubia* Mc. Vaugh) for antihyperglycemia, antihypertension, antimicrobial properties and cellular rejuvenation." *Food Res. Int.* 2015; 77(Part 2): 194–203.

Kaneshima T, et al. "Antimicrobial constituents of peel and seeds of camu camu (*Myrciaria dubia*)." *Biosci. Biotechnol. Biochem.* 2017 Aug; 81(8): 1461–1465.

Lopez-Mata, A. "Antibacterial effect of the juice of *Myrciaria dubia, Citrus grande* and *Citrus reticula* on *Escherichia coli* and *Salmonella tiphy.*" *CIENTIFI-K.* 2017; 5(1): 87–92.

Mirzale, S., et al. "Investigation for antimicrobial resistance-modulating activity of diethyl malate and 1-methyl malate against beta-lactamase class A from

Bacillus licheniformis by molecular dynamics, *in vitro* and *in vivo* studies." *J. Biomol. Struct. Dyn.* 2015; 33(5): 1016–26.

Mori, T., et al. "Antimicrobial effect of *Myrciaria dubia* (camu camu) and *Cyperus luzulae* (piri piri) on pathogenic microorganisms." 2016; *Conoc. Amaz.* 4: 49–57.

Moromi, H., "Effectiveness *in vitro* and *in vivo* of a *Myrciaria dubia* based mouthwash on important oral bacteria." *Theorema.* 2014 Jun; 1(1): 83–92.

Myoda, T., et al. "Antioxidative and antimicrobial potential of residues of camu camu juice production." *J. Food. Agricult. Environ.* 2010; 8: 304–307.

Pardo-Aldalve, K., et al. *"Myrciaria dubia*: its potential as adjunct in the treatment of periodontal disease." *Revista Cubana.* 2019; 56(4): e1779.

Pardo-Aldave, K., "Antimicrobial activity *in vitro* of camu camu (*Myrciaria dubia*) against oral microorganisms: A systematic review." *Rev. Peru Med. Exp. Salud Publica.* 2019 Oct–Dec; 36(4): 573–582.

Roumy, V., et al. "Plant therapy in the Peruvian Amazon (Loreto) in case of infectious diseases and its antimicrobial evaluation." *J. Ethnopharmacol.* 2020 Mar; 249: 112411.

Saldarriaga-Mostacero, E. "*In vitro* antibacterial effect of the ethanol extract of *Myrciaria dubia* (camu camu) on *Streptococcus mutans*." Thesis 2017. National University of Trujillo, School of Dentistry. Trujillo, Peru.

Varela-Lopez, A., et al. "Non-nutrient, natural, occurring phenolic compounds with antioxidant activity for the prevention and treatment of periodontal diseases." *Antioxidants.* 2015; 4(3): 447-81.

Anti-Obesity and Antidiabetic Actions

Ahangarpour, A., et al. "The antidiabetic and antioxidant properties of some phenolic phytochemicals: A review study." *Diabetes Metab. Syndr.* 2019 Jan–Feb; 13(1): 854–857.

Amin, M., et al. "Estimation of ellagic acid and/or repaglinide effects on insulin signaling, oxidative stress, and inflammatory mediators of liver, pancreas, adipose tissue, and brain in insulin resistant/type 2 diabetic rats." *Appl. Physiol. Nutr. Metab.* 2017 Feb; 42(2): 181–192.

Anhe. F., et al. "Treatment with camu camu (*Myrciaria dubia*) prevents obesity by altering the gut microbiota and increasing energy expenditure in diet-induced obese mice." *Gut.* 2018 Jul: 68: 453–464.

Balisteiro, D., et al. "Effect of clarified Brazilian native fruit juices on postprandial glycemia in healthy subjects." *Food Res. Int.* 2017; 100: 196–203.

Donado-Pestana, C., et al. "Polyphenols from Brazilian native *Myrtaceae* fruits

References

and their potential health benefits against obesity and its associated complications." *Curr. Opin. Food Sci.* 2018; 19: 42–49.

Fujita, A., et al. "Evaluation of phenolic-linked bioactives of camu camu (*Myrciaria dubia* Mc. Vaugh) for antihyperglycemia, antihypertension, antimicrobial properties and cellular rejuvenation." *Food Res. Int.* 2015; 77(Part 2): 194–203.

Goncalves, A., et al. "Chemical composition and antioxidant/ antidiabetic potential of Brazilian native fruits and commercial frozen pulps." *J. Agric. Food Chem.* 2010; 58: 4666–4674.

Goncalves, A., et al. "Frozen pulp extracts of camu camu (*Myrciaria dubia* McVaugh) attenuate the hyperlipidemia and lipid peroxidation of type 1 diabetic rats. *Food Res. Int.* 2014 Oct; 64: 1–8.

Kim, K., et al. "Betulinic acid inhibits high-fat diet-induced obesity and improves energy balance by activating AMPK." *Nutr. Metab. Cardiovasc. Dis.* 2019 Apr; 29(4): 409–420.

Nascimento, O., et al. "Effects of diet supplementation with camu camu (*Myrciaria dubia* HBK McVaugh) fruit in a rat model of diet-induced obesity." *An. Acad. Bras. Cienc.* 2013 Mar; 85(1): 355–63.

Wang, L., et al. "Ellagic acid promotes browning of white adipose tissues in high-fat diet-induced obesity in rats through suppressing white adipocyte maintaining genes." *Endocr. J.* 2019 Oct; 66(10): 923–936.

Vargas, B., et al. "Effect of camu camu capsules on blood glucose and lipid profile of healthy adults." *Rev. Cubana Plantas Med.* 2015; 20: 48–61.

Wang, S., et al. "Novel insights of dietary polyphenols and obesity." *J. Nutr. Biochem.* 2014 Jan; 25(1): 1–18.

Antioxidant Actions

Akter, M., et al. "Nutritional compositions and health promoting phytochemicals of camu camu (*Myrciaria dubia*) fruit: a review." *Food Res. Int.* 2011; 44: 1728–1732.

Arellano-Acuna, E., et al. "Camu camu (*Myrciaria dubia*): Tropical fruit of excellent functional properties that help to improve the quality of life." *Sci. Agropecuaria.* 2016; 7(4): 433–443.

Avila-Sosa, R., et al. "Antioxidant properties of Amazonian fruits: a mini review of *in vivo* and *in vitro* studies." *Oxidat. Med. Cell. Longev.* 2019; 2019: 8204129.

Azevedo, L., et al. "Camu camu (*Myrciaria dubia*) from commercial cultivation has higher levels of bioactive compounds than native cultivation (Amazon Forest) and presents antimutagenic effects *in vivo*." *J. Sci. Food Agric.* 2019 Jan; 99(2): 624–631.

Chirinos, R., "Antioxidant compounds and antioxidant capacity of Peruvian camu camu (*Myrciara dubia* [H.B.K.] McVaugh) fruit at different maturity stages." *Food Chem.* 2010; 120: 1019–1024.

da Silva, F., et al. "Antigenotoxic effect of acute, subacute and chronic treatments with Amazonian camu camu (*Myrciaria dubia*) juice on mice blood cells." *Food Chem. Toxicol.* 2012 Jul; 50(7): 2275–81.

de Carvalho-Silva L., et al. "Antiproliferative, antimutagenic and antioxidant activities of a Brazilian tropical fruit juice." *Food Sci. Technol.* 2014; 59: 1319–1324.

Fidelis, M., et al. "*In vitro* antioxidant and antihypertensive compounds from camu camu (*Myrciaria dubia* McVaugh, Myrtaceae) seed coat: A multivariate structure-activity study." *Food Chem. Toxicol.* 2018 Oct; 120: 479–490.

Fracassetti, D., et al. "Ellagic acid derivatives, ellagitannins, proanthocyanidins and other phenolics, vitamin C and antioxidant capacity of two powder products from camu camu fruit (*Myrciaria dubia*)." *Food Chem.* 2013 Aug; 139(1-4): 578–88.

Franco, M., et al. "Volatile composition of some Brazilian fruits: umbu-caja (*Spondias citherea*), camu camu (*Myrciaria dubia*), Araca-boi (*Eugenia stipitata*), and Cupuacu (*Theobroma grandiflorum*)." *J. Agric. Food Chem.* 2000; 48(4): 1263–5.

Fujita, A., et al. "Evaluation of phenolic-linked bioactives of camu camu (*Myrciaria dubia* Mc. Vaugh) for antihyperglycemia, antihypertension, antimicrobial properties and cellular rejuvenation." *Food Res. Int.* 2015; 77(Part 2): 194–203.

Genovese, M., et al. "Bioactive compounds and antioxidant capacity of exotic fruits and commercial frozen pulps from Brazil." *Food Sci. Technol. Int.* 2008; 14: 207–214.

Goncalves, A., et al. "Chemical composition and antioxidant/antidiabetic potential of Brazilian native fruits and commercial frozen pulps." *J. Agric. Food Chem.* 2010; 58: 4666–4674.

Inoue, T., et al. "Tropical fruit camu camu (*Myrciaria dubia*) has anti-oxidative and anti-inflammatory properties." *J. Cardiol.* 2008 Oct; 52(2): 127–32.

Ju, A., et al. "Development of teff starch films containing camu camu (*Myrciaria dubia* Mc. Vaugh) extract as an antioxidant packaging material." *Indus. Crop. Prod.* 2019 Dec; 141: 11137.

Kaneshima, T., et al. "Antioxidant activity of C-Glycosidic ellagitannins from the seeds and peel of camu camu (*Myrciaria dubia*)." *Food Sci. Technol.* 2016; 69: 76–81.

Langley, P., et al. "Antioxidant and associated capacities of camu camu (*Myrciaria dubia*): a systematic review." *J. Altern. Complement. Med.* 2015 Jan; 21(1): 8–14.

References

Pereira, A., et al. "Effect of antioxidant potential of tropical fruit juices on antioxidant enzyme profiles and lipid peroxidation in rats." *Food Chem.* 2014; 157: 179-185.

Myoda, T., et al. "Antioxidative and antimicrobial potential of residues of camu camu juice production." *J. Food. Agricult. Environ.* 2010; 8: 304–307.

Neri-Numa, I., et al. "Small Brazilian wild fruits: Nutrients, bioactive compounds, health-promotion properties and commercial interest." *Food Res. Int.* 2018 Jan; 103: 345–360.

Reynertson, K., et al. "Quantitative analysis of antiradical [antioxidant] phenolic constituents from fourteen edible *Myrtaceae* fruits." *Food Chem.* 2008; 109(4): 883–890.

Rufino, M., et al. "Free radical scavenging behavior of ten exotic tropical fruits extracts." *Food Res. Int.* 2011: 44: 2072–2075.

Rufino, M., et al. "Bioactive compounds and antioxidant capacities of 18 non-traditional tropical fruits from Brazil." *Food Chem.* 2010; 12(4): 996-1002.

Rodrigues, R., et al. "Antioxidant capacity of camu camu [*Myrciaria dubia* (H.B.K.) McVaugh] pulp." *Ernahrung. Nutr.* 2006; 30: 357–362.

Solis, V., et al. "Antioxidant activity from pulp, peel and seed of camu camu (*Myrciaria dubia* H.B.K)." *Rev. Soc. Quim. Peru.* 2009; 75: 293–299.

Sotero, V., et al. "Evaluation of the antioxidant activity of the pulp, peel and seed of camu camu fruit (*Myrciaria dubia* H.B.K.)." *Revista Soc. Chem. Peru.* 2009; 75(3): 293–299.

Villanueva-Tiburcio, J., et al. "Anthocyanins, ascorbic acid, total polyphenols and antioxidant activity in camu camu peel (*Myrciaria dubia* (H.B.K) McVaugh)." *Food Sci. Technol. Camp.* 2010; 30: 151–160.

Zanatta, C., et al. "Determination of anthocyanins from camu camu (*Myrciaria dubia*) by HPLC-PDA, HPLC-MS, and NMR." *J. Agric. Food Chem.* 2005 Nov; 53(24): 9531–5.

Zanatta, C., et al. "Carotenoid composition from the Brazilian tropical fruit camu–camu (*Myrciaria dubia*)." *Food Chem.* 2007; 4: 1526–1532.

Zeb, A., "Ellagic acid in suppressing *in vivo* and *in vitro* oxidative stresses." *Mol. Cell Biochem.* 2018 Nov; 448(1-2): 27–41.

Cellular-Protective Antioxidant Actions

Akachi, T., et al. "L-methylmalate from camu camu (*Myrciaria dubia*) suppressed D-galactosamine-induced liver injury in rats." *Biosci. Biotechnol. Biochem.* 2010; 74(3): 573–8.

Azevedo, J., et al. "Neuroprotective effects of dried camu camu (*Myrciaria dubia* HBK McVaugh) residue in *C. elegans*." *Food Res. Intl.* 2015 Jul; 73: 135–141.

Becerra, K., et al. "Nephroprotective effect of camu camu (*Myrciaria dubia*) in a model of nephrotoxicity induced by Gentamicin in rats." *Rev. Chil. Nutr.* 2019 Jun; 46(3): 303–307.

Chakraborty, S., et al. "Oxidative stress mechanisms underlying Parkinson's Disease-associated neurodegeneration in *C. elegans*." *Int. J. Mol. Sci.* 2013; 14: 23103–23128.

da Silva, F., et al. "Antigenotoxic and antimutagenic effects of *Myrciaria dubia* juice in mice submitted to ethanol 28-day treatment." *J. Toxicol. Environ. Health A.* 2019; 82(17): 956–968.

Doroteo, V., et al. "Phenolic compounds and antioxidant, antielastase, anticollagenase and photoprotective *in vitro* activities of *Myrciaria dubia* (camu camu) and *Caesalpinia spinosa* (tara)." *Rev. Soc. Quim. Peru.* 2012; 78(4): 254–263.

Garcia-Nino, W., et al. "Ellagic acid: Pharmacological activities and molecular mechanisms involved in liver protection." *Pharmacol. Res.* 2015 Jul; 97: 84–103.

Inocente-Camones, M., et al. "Antioxidant activity and photoprotective *in vitro* of lotion and gel processed with extract stabilized of camu camu (*Myrciaria dubia* Kunth)." *Rev. Soc. Quim. Peru.* 2014; 80(1): 65–77.

Cancer-Preventative Actions

Alvis, R. "Detection of the antimutagenic effect of the aqueous extract of the fruit of *Myrciaria dubia* H. B. K. Mc Vaugh "camu camu", using the *in vivo* micronucleus test." 2010 Thesis. Universidad Nacional Mayor de San Marcos. Lima, Peru.

Asmat-Aguirre, S. "Effect of *Myrciaria dubia* (H.B.K) Mc Vaugh fruit on induced colorectal cancer in *Rattus norvegicus* var. Albinus." Thesis 2017. National University of Trujillo, School of Pharmacy and Biochemistry, Trujillo, Peru.

Azevedo, L., et al. "Camu camu (*Myrciaria dubia*) from commercial cultivation has higher levels of bioactive compounds than native cultivation (Amazon Forest) and presents antimutagenic effects *in vivo*." *J. Sci. Food Agric.* 2019 Jan; 99(2): 624–631.

Ceci, C., et al. "Experimental evidence of the antitumor, antimetastatic and antiangiogenic activity of ellagic acid." *Nutrients.* 2018 Nov 14; 10(11).

da Silva, F., et al. "Antigenotoxic and antimutagenic effects of *Myrciaria dubia* juice in mice submitted to ethanol 28-day treatment." *J. Toxicol. Environ. Health A.* 2019; 82(17): 956–968.

de Carvalho-Silva, L., et al. "Antiproliferative, antimutagenic and antioxidant activities of a Brazilian tropical fruit juice." *Food Sci. Technol.* 2014; 59: 1319–1324.

References

Gheorgheosu, D., et al. "Betulinic acid as a potent and complex antitumor phytochemical: A minireview." *Anticancer Agents Med. Chem.* 2014; 14(7): 936–45.

Gutierrez, J. "Protective ability of *Myrciaria dubia* "camu camu" against oxidative stress-induced genetic damage, evaluated *in vitro*, in the "Chinese hamster" ovary cell line *Cricetulus griseus* and *in vivo Drosophila melanogaster* "fruit fly."" 2007 Doctoral Thesis. Universidad Nacional de Trujillo. Trujillo, Peru.

Khuda-Bukhsh, A., et al. "Molecular approaches toward targeted cancer prevention with some food plants and their products: inflammatory and other signal pathways." *Nutr. Cancer.* 2014; 66(2): 194–205.

Sanchez, H. "Evaluation of the antioxidant capacity, phenolic compounds and antimutagenic activity of the extracts of camu camu (*Myrciaria dubia*) and Yacón (*Smallanthus sonchifolius*)." 2010 Thesis. Universidad Nacional Agraria La Molina. Lima, Peru.

Shakeri, A., et al. "Ellagic Acid: A logical lead for drug development?" *Curr. Pharm. Des.* 2018; 24(2): 106–122.

Zhang, H., et al. "Research progress on the anticarcinogenic actions and mechanisms of ellagic acid." *Cancer Biol. Med.* 2014 Jun; 11(2): 92–100.

Cholesterol-Lowering Actions

Goncalves, A., et al. "Frozen pulp extracts of camu camu (*Myrciaria dubia* McVaugh) attenuate the hyperlipidemia and lipid peroxidation of type 1 diabetic rats. *Food Res. Int.* 2014 Oct; 64: 1–8.

Nascimento, O., et al. "Effects of diet supplementation with camu camu (*Myrciaria dubia* HBK McVaugh) fruit in a rat model of diet-induced obesity." *An. Acad. Bras. Cienc.* 2013 Mar; 85(1): 355–63.

Schwertz, M., et al. "Hypolipidemic effect of camu camu juice in rats." *Rev. Nutr.* 2012; 25: 35–44.

Donado-Pestana, C., et al. "Polyphenols from Brazilian native *Myrtaceae* fruits and their potential health benefits against obesity and its associated complications." *Curr. Opin. Food Sci.* 2018; 19: 42–49.

Goncalves, F. "Effect of camu camu juice (*Myrciaria dubia* (Kunth) McVaugh) on serum cholesterol, triglyceride and glucose levels in adults." 2012 Dissertation. Post-Graduate Pharmaceutical Sciences in Food Science. Universidade Federal do Amazonas, Manaus, Brazil.

Pereira, A., et al. "Effect of antioxidant potential of tropical fruit juices on antioxidant enzyme profiles and lipid peroxidation in rats." *Food Chem.* 2014; 157: 179–185.

Vargas, B., et al. "Effect of camu camu capsules on blood glucose and lipid profile of healthy adults." *Rev. Cubana Plantas Med.* 2015; 20: 48–61.

Fertility Enhancement Actions

Torres, L., et al. *"Myrciaria dubia* "camu camu" flour as a magnetoprotector in male mouse infertility." *Bioelectromagnetics.* 2019 Feb; 40(2): 91–103.

Gonzales, G., et al. "The transillumination technique as a method for the assessment of spermatogenesis using medicinal plants: the effect of extracts of black maca (*Lepidium meyenii*) and camu camu (*Myrciaria dubia*) on stages of the spermatogenic cycle in male rats." *Toxicol. Mech. Methods.* 2013 Oct; 23(8): 559–65.

Silva, E., et al. "(In)Fertility and oxidative stress: New insights into novel redox mechanisms controlling fundamental reproductive processes." *Oxid. Med. Cell. Longev.* 2020 Jan 21; 2020: 4674896

Immune Stimulant Actions

Macedo, R., and Mendoza J. "Immunostimulant activity of the fruit *Myrciaria dubia* H.B.K. McVaugh "camu camu," in Holtzman albino white rats." Thesis 2015. Universidad Nacional de la Amazonía Peruana. Iquitos, Peru.

Yunis-Aguinaga, J., et al. "Dietary camu camu, *Myrciaria dubia*, enhances immunological response in Nile tilapia." *Fish Shellf. Immunol.* 2016; 58: 284–291.

Chapter 7. A Consumer Guide for Camu Camu

Non-Toxic Effect

da Silva, F., et al. "Antigenotoxic effect of acute, subacute and chronic treatments with Amazonian camu camu (*Myrciaria dubia*) juice on mice blood cells." *Food Chem. Toxicol.* 2012; 50: 2275–2281.

Castro, L, et al. "Evaluation of the mutagenic effect of the juice of the *Myrciaria* fruit H.B.K. (McVaugh) (CAMU CAMU) by means of a micronucleus test on the bone marrow of mice." [Poster Abstract]. Presented at the 57th Congresso Brasileiro de Genetica, Aguas de Lindoia, Brasil, August 30–September 2, 2011.

Research on Camu Camu Seeds

Carmo, M., et al. "Hydroalcoholic *Myrciaria dubia* (camu camu) seed extracts prevent chromosome damage and act as antioxidant and cytotoxic agents." *Food Res. Int.* 2019 Nov; 125: 108551.

Conceicao, N., et al. "By-products of camu camu [*Myrciaria dubia* (Kunth) McVaugh] as promising sources of bioactive high added-value food ingredients: functionalization of yogurts. *Molecules.* 2019 Dec 24; 25(1).

Fidelis, M., et al. "Camu camu seed (*Myrciaria dubia*)–From side stream to an antioxidant, antihyperglycemic, antiproliferative, antimicrobial, antihemolytic, anti-inflammatory, and antihypertensive ingredient." *Food Chem.* 2020 Apr; 310: 125909.

References

Fidelis, M., et al. "*In vitro* antioxidant and antihypertensive compounds from camu camu (*Myrciaria dubia* McVaugh, Myrtaceae) seed coat: A multivariate structure-activity study." *Food Chem. Toxicol.* 2018 Oct; 120: 479–490.

Kaneshima, T., et al. "Antimicrobial constituents of peel and seeds of camu camu (*Myrciaria dubia*)." *Biosci. Biotechnol. Biochem.* 2017 Aug; 81(8): 1461–1465.

Kaneshima, T., et al. "Antioxidant activity of C-Glycosidic ellagitannins from the seeds and peel of camu camu (*Myrciaria dubia).*" *Food Sci. Technol.* 2016; 69: 76–81.

Yazawa, K., et al. "Anti-inflammatory effects of seeds of the tropical fruit camu camu (*Myrciaria dubia*)." *J. Nutr. Sci. Vitaminol.* 2011; 57(1): 104–7.

Manufacturing Methods:

Azevedo, J., et al. "Dried camu camu (*Myrciaria dubia* H.B.K. McVaugh) industrial residue: A bioactive-rich Amazonian powder with functional attributes." *Food Res. Int.* 2014; 62: 934–940.

Brizzolari, A., et al. "Antioxidant capacity and heat damage of powder products from South American plants with functional properties." *Ital. J. Food Sci.* 2019 May; 31(4): 731–748.

Castro, J., et al. "Variation of the contents of vitamin C and anthocyanins in *Myrciaria dubia* "camu camu." *Rev. Soc. Chem. Peru.* 2013; 79(4): 319–330.

Conceiaco, N., et al. "By products of camu camu [*Myrciaria dubia* (Kunth) McVaugh] as promising sources of bioactive high added-value food ingredients: functionalization of yogurts." *Molecules.* 2019 Dec 24; 25(1).

Cunha-Santos, E., et al. "Vitamin C in camu camu [*Myrciaria dubia* (H.B.K.) McVaugh]: evaluation of extraction and analytical methods." *Food. Res. Int.* 2019 Jan; 115: 160–166.

Dib Taxi, C., et al. "Study of the microencapsulation of camu camu (*Myrciaria dubia*) juice." *J. Microencapsul.* 2003 Jul–Aug; 20(4): 443–8.

Fidelis, M., et al. "From byproduct to a functional ingredient: Camu camu (*Myrciaria dubia*) seed extract as an antioxidant agent in a yogurt model." *J. Dairy Sci.* 2020 Feb; 103(2): 1131–1140.

Fracassetti, D., et al. "Ellagic acid derivatives, ellagitannins, proanthocyanidins and other phenolics, vitamin C and antioxidant capacity of two powder products from camu camu fruit (*Myrciaria dubia*)." *Food Chem.* 2013 Aug; 139(1-4): 578–88.

Fujita, A., et al. "Effects of spray-drying parameters on *in vitro* functional properties of camu camu (*Myrciaria dubia* Mc. Vaugh): A typical Amazonian fruit." *J. Food Sci.* 2017 May; 82(5): 1083–1091.

Camu Camu

Fujita, A., et al. "Evaluation of phenolic-linked bioactives of camu camu (*Myrciaria dubia* Mc. Vaugh) for antihyperglycemia, antihypertension, antimicrobial properties and cellular rejuvenation." *Food Res. Int.* 2015; 77(Part 2): 194–203.

Fujita, A., et al. "Improving anti-hyperglycemic and anti-hypertensive properties of camu camu (*Myriciaria dubia* Mc. Vaugh) using lactic acid bacterial fermentation." *Process Biochem.* 2017; 59: 133–140.

Justi, K., et al. "Nutritional composition and vitamin C stability in stored camu camu (*Myrciaria dubia*) pulp." *Arch. Latinoam. Nutr.* 2000 Dec; 50(4): 405–8.

Kaneshima, T., et al. "Antioxidative constituents in camu camu fruit juice residue." *Food Sci. Technol. Res.* 2013; 19(2): 223–8.

Neves, L., et al. "Post-harvest nutraceutical behaviour during ripening and senescence of 8 highly perishable fruit species from the northern Brazilian Amazon region." *Food Chem.* 2015; 174: 188–196.

Padilha, C., "Recovery of polyphenols from camu camu (*Myrciaria dubia* H.B.K. McVaugh) depulping residue by cloud point extraction." *Chin. J. Chem. Eng.* 2018; 26: 2471–2476.

Padilha, C., et al. "Enhancing the recovery and concentration of polyphenols from camu camu (*Myrciaria dubia* H.B.K. McVaugh) by aqueous two-phase flotation and scale-up process." *Separation Sci. Tech.* 2018; 53: 1–10.

Rodrigues, L, et al. "Camu camu bioactive compounds extraction by ecofriendly sequential processes (ultrasound assisted extraction and reverse osmosis)." *Ultrason. Sonochem.* 2020 Jun; 64: 105017.

Wulitzer, N., et al. "Tropical fruit juice: effect of thermal treatment and storage time on sensory and functional properties." *J. Food Sci. Technol.* 2019 Dec; 56(12): 5184–5193.

Zillo, R., et al. "Camu camu harvested with reddish-green peel preserves its physicochemical characteristics and antioxidant compounds during cold storage." *Braz. J. Food Technol.* 2019; 22: e2017060.

About the Author

Leslie Taylor is one of the world's leading experts on rainforest medicinal plants. She founded, managed, and directed the Raintree group of companies from 1995 to 2012, and was a leader in creating a worldwide market for the important medicinal plants of the Amazon rainforest.

Having survived a rare form of leukemia only because of alternative health and herbal medicine, Leslie has been researching, studying, and documenting alternative healing modalities—including herbal medicine—for more than thirty years. A dedicated herbalist and naturopath, she developed many herbal formulas and remedies for her companies, for practitioners, and for individuals needing help. In 1995, while researching alternative AIDS and cancer therapies in Europe, Leslie became aware of a medicinal plant from the Peruvian rainforest called cat's claw. This research took her to the Peruvian rainforest to gain firsthand knowledge about this new medicinal plant. Upon her return, she founded Raintree Nutrition, Inc., to make this important rainforest medicinal plant and others available in the United States.

After that first trip, Leslie returned to the Amazon numerous times, continuing to research and document more rainforest medicinal plants. In these endeavors, she worked directly with indigenous Indian shamans and healers, learning about their use of healing plants, as well as with indigenous tribal communities and other rainforest communities. She also worked with phytochemists, botanists, ethnobotanists, researchers, and alternative and integrative health practitioners to document, research, test, and validate rainforest medicinal plants.

In 2012, with many other companies selling the rainforest plants that she had introduced to the United States, she decided to close her business and naturopathic practice and devote herself to educating people about the benefits of medicinal plants. She freely shared all her proprietary formulas by posting them on the Raintree website so that anyone can make and use them.

Now, Leslie Taylor remains a trusted source of factual information about rainforest medicinal plants and continues to update the Tropical Plant Database for these purposes. A practicing board certified naturopath for many years (now retired), she has lectured and taught classes in naturopathic medicine, herbal medicine, and ethnobotany, as well as environmental and sustainability issues in the Amazon rainforest. She is the author of *Herbal Secrets of the Rainforest* and of the best-selling *The Healing Power of Rainforest Herbs*, as well as the highly popular and extensively referenced Raintree Tropical Plant Database (http://www.rain-tree.com/plants.htm), which has been online since 1996.

More information about Leslie Taylor and her other books can be found at http://rain-tree.com/author.htm and on her Amazon Author Page. She also has a personal blog where you can ask questions and share your results using camu camu with others at https://leslie-taylor-raintree.blogspot.com.